Intermittent Fasting for Women

An Effective Step by step Guide to a Fasting Diet for Women with a Scientific Approach Including Keto Fast Diet

by

Emma Lyron

Disclaimer Notice

Please note the information contained in this document is for educational and entertainment purposes only. All effort has been executed to present accurate, up to date, and reliable, complete information. No warranties of any kind are declared or implied. Readers acknowledge that the author is not engaging in the rendering of legal, financial, medical, or professional advice. The content in this book has been derived from various sources. Please consult a licensed professional before attempting any techniques outlined in this book.

By reading this document, the reader agrees that under no circumstances is the author responsible for any losses, direct or indirect, which are incurred as a result of the use of the information contained in this document, including, but not limited to, — errors, omissions, or inaccuracies.

or monetary loss due to the information contained in this book. Either directly or indirectly. You are responsible for your own choices, actions, and results.

Table of Contents

Introduction

Dieting is complicated! There are numerous options available that it can sometimes feel overwhelming don't even know where to start out. And maybe you've tried them all— the diet, the Atkins diet, the Paleo diet— and none of them succeeded, so you want to undertake something new.

It's here where intermittent fasting fits in. It's one of the most well-liked new ways and for an excellent reason to lose weight! It isn't a diet; it's an eating style. It is thanks to planning your meals so as to urge the foremost out of them.

Fasting is an old custom practiced by various nationalities and cultures in early times. Beneficial intermittent fasts for solving problems with excessive fat were studied as early as 1915. This captured the eye of the medical world in the mid-1900s after Bloom and the company made a viable report. Intermittent fasts, also referred to as IF, were in the range of 1 to 14 days in these studies.

This interest started being shared in bulletins, which reminded people to remember and be careful about the utilization of intermittent fasting without advice from a medical professional.

The latest quite intermittent fasting is additionally referred to as the 5:2 Diet, which started in Britain several years ago.

There is a spread of intermittent fasting, which may be found in religious traditions everywhere in the world. Samples of religious fasting include Vrata, Ramadan, Christian Fasting, and lots of more. Some religious fasting customs only take staying faraway from certain foods, while others, like Yom Kippur, take not eating food for a quick period and might end in unnoticeable effects on an individual's BMI.

Choosing the intermittent fasting approach has many benefits, including:

- It has been scientifically proven to assist you in reducing and fat in the stomach.
- It can improve your health, and it can assist cure diseases like diabetes and heart attacks.
- It can help prevent infections and assist you at the end of the day.
- It keeps the brain is basically healthy.
- It can allow you to measure length.

Of course, in this text, we'll enter more depth on how intermittent fasting will assist you in turning your life around. Actually, on the market, you'll not be ready to find a more comprehensive guide. It not only addresses the simplest diets to follow, but it'll also guarantee that you simply are fully equipped with tools to regulate your pace and keeping you safe in the process.

In addition to all or any this, you'll even be ready to see a variety of scientific studies performed in reference to intermittent fasting—showing that the wellbeing, weight, and brain effects are real. Once you've got checked out just what was being tried for fasting, you'll be more persuaded than ever before. Regardless of the ultimate goal is, you will see how fasting will achieve it.

It's literally all you would like, beat one place. Once you finish reading, you will have all you would like to urge you started with the right intermittent fasting diet for you—so don't put it off anymore; let's continue!

Developing a Healthy Lifestyle Both Mentally and Physically

Having an unhealthy lifestyle can cause many unwanted physical and mental problems. Most people do not realize what proportion strain is on your mind and body once you do not have the right level of hormones and vitamins in your body, which accompanies a healthy lifestyle.

Many people think these diseases and sicknesses are inherited, which there's nothing they will do to stop or heal them. This is often not true in most cases! Watching what you eat and getting the right amount of exercise will cause you to feel far better than taking some quite pill for your problem. For instance, someone with high blood pressure or high sugar can take medications which will help them to regulate their disease but what many of them do not know is that if they did regular cardiovascular exercise and ate healthier foods, they probably wouldn't even need to take the medications and would also feel great!

Most people want to measure a healthy lifestyle, but they do not have the right tools to urge started. They also don't maintain the self-motivation it takes to be persistent enough to stay to a healthy living pattern. The primary thing to do is to make a decision about what your goals are. Once you've got come up together with your goals, then you've got accomplished the primary step to your healthy lifestyle!

What Does It Mean to possess A Healthy Body?

According to David Kirsch, if the mind isn't healthy, you'll never get a sound body.

Since the body takes us everywhere we would like to travel; it's therefore imperative that the body is ready to move with ease. All organs, joints, and muscles must perform well on a day to day to make a move simple and stylish. Once you have a healthy body, you are feeling light and energetic; and you are doing not tire easily. Also, there's a glow a healthy body radiates. A healthy body doesn't concede easily to weather, virus, or heat. A healthy body can support and avoid the expansion of diseases.

Do not equate health with exercise. These are two very different aspects of well-being. One is not the same because the other. Although it's possible to be healthy and not fit and the other way around, we'll aspire for a healthy and fit body's equilibrium.

It's better to urge a fit body because it is easy and more measurable. The philosophy of fitness produces egotism that relies on the trivial. We're so focused on the surface; we lose sight of what is happening inside. This is often why, while the culture of exercise is increasing, we are still facing a plague of health.

The reality is that health and what it entails to be healthy remains not fully understood. We function in a mode of survival, functioning in an inadequate way, embracing mediocrity.

There's such a lot of material out there that you simply will quickly stray and frustrated. We're just shocked by overloading details and doing nothing. And, without the right understanding, we follow trends. We've forgotten the link to our physical body, and that we do not know the way to help it.

Putting Your Mental State In Shape As You Diet

Losing weight and happening a diet is often quite challenging! As someone who has lost over 50 pounds, I will be able to share a touch of my "dieting wisdom" with you.

- Throw out that scale! In fact, we all want to stay track of our progress, but stepping thereon scale every day is not the thanks to roll in the hay. In fact, it can keep us from that specialize in what we actually should be that specialize in. A preoccupation with what the size reads can cause us to become dependent and depressed. Instead, keep close attention to how you feel - lack of energy and tiredness might be a sign that you simply are failing to lose weight in the healthiest way. On the other hand, increased energy might be a symbol that you simply are getting healthier. Specialize in what your body tells you--monitor how clothes are fitting you. This is often a way more positive way of monitoring your weight loss. Save the size for normal doctor's checkups or occasional, periodic use.

- Set realistic goals. Trying to "lose weight fast" is usually times not only impractical but also dangerous. Set goals that you simply know are often feasibly integrated into your daily routine (more of goal setting in subsequent chapters). Not only are quick weight loss attempts often difficult to take care of, but they will even be hazardous to your health-- causing you to ruin your metabolism and rapidly regain the load as soon as you stop your diet.

- Expect fallbacks. We all have our bad days. Being hard on yourself for breaking your diet and falling back on your weight goals is a component of the process! Frustration can make it even harder to urge back on target. Instead, anticipate and choose ways in which you'll be more dedicated to your goals. Keeping a journal can help.

- Praise yourself often. Remember, attaining your weight goals is simply the maximum amount of a process because it may be a physical one. For this reason, it's important to stay motivated. Consider ways to positively reward yourself. For example: get your nails done or have a guys-only night out. There are all types of the way to pamper yourself without spending an excessive amount of money. Be creative!

- Be open together with your doctor. If you're struggling in achieving your goals, don't keep trying to do it alone! Contact your doctor. He/she could also be ready to assist you in customizing your goals or refer you to a nutritionist or other professional trained to assist patients mentally and physically stay track when losing weight.

Above all, remember that losing weight doesn't mean foregoing fun and ignoring what your mind and emotions tell you. In fact, listening to your psychological state can ultimately mean much better results. Ditch the size, be realistic, reward yourself, and, if needed, seek professional assistance. With the right mindset, you'll already be on your thanks to reaching your weight loss goals!

Staying Motivated

Motivation is the key to continuing and sticking to the idea of losing weight. Most of the people who start a diet or exercise routine have problems staying motivated to continue with it and ultimately quit. Supported the statistics from the CDC for 2007-2008, 34% of yank adults are overweight. This is often up from the previous stats from 2005-2006 of 32.7%. These statistics are only a glimpse at the overwhelming problem of obesity in America.

Thousands of individuals start a diet or weight loss routine per annum; however, the people that stick with their goals are minimal. Motivation plays an enormous role in whether someone will reach his or her weight loss goals. People that are overweight or obese usually know that their health is suffering from their weight; however, they do not care or don't think that they will do anything about it. Most of the time, people make excuses for not starting a workout routine, or they're just lazy to truly roll in the hay. Although the intention of becoming healthier may be a great notion, it perils to match to the particular act of dieting or losing weight.

Using motivational tools can't only keep you on the right path of becoming a healthier person but can get you to your goal weight in the acceptable time-frame. Losing weight isn't easy. People that think like this are sure to hand over, quit or relapse quicker. Unfortunately, weight loss television shows give people that are overweight an inaccurate depiction of how easy it's to reduce. In our society, we are bombarded with unhealthy options, which will make losing weight harder. Also, the limit of your time, availability, and options can limit one's ability to make healthy choices ultimately, though it's up to you to make a choice and determination to realize your weight loss goals.

Surround yourself with motivation. This includes having encouraging people in your family, at work, or in your group of friends. These people will push you to continue on. You'll want to incorporate your family into your new lifestyle. Or workout every day with a lover who wants to reduce too. Put encouraging words or phrases in your calendar, on your bulletin board, or anywhere that you simply will see it. These words can inspire you to stay going. Create a dream board. Put pictures or images of things that you simply want to do, how you would like to seem, or overall goals that you simply want to realize. Put it somewhere you'll see it every day; that way, once you check it out, you'll want to stay going. Read stories, blogs, or watch videos of other people's transformations. Although not everyone can get the experience of being on "The Biggest Loser," but there are contestants whose stories have inspired and created a sequence reaction causing thousands to urge up and reduce. Reward yourself. Most rewards are related to food; however, a gift is often in the sort of a replacement shirt, a replacement phone, or maybe a replacement piece of jewelry. Rewards are often set at the time once you set your goals or decided upon whenever you reach your goal. Either way, it'll cause you to feel good about what you're doing and motivate you to stay going.

The main point to recollect is that the sole thanks to getting your healthy lifestyle are to stay on trying a day. Eventually, your lifestyle changes become a habit . In other words, after you become familiar with your lifestyle changes, they're going to become how of life rather than something you're making yourself do to feel good.

What Is Intermittent Fasting?

Fasting is the abstention process of food and drink for a particular amount of your time. A process of feeding and fasting is understood as intermittent fasting (IF). It is so common because it doesn't decide such a lot what to eat–eliminating many people that are on strict diets or do not like those foods–it's more focused on when to eat.

There's a lot of various ways you'll do that easily–there's nothing in stone about it, which suggests you'll work it into your lifestyle anyway. We're getting to check out some explanations of how you'll bring this into your life, and what quite things you are going to take to do and obtain the foremost of your food, later in this book. Let's check out how intermittent fasting works for now.

Intermittent fasting, as has already been said, isn't a diet. It is a way people are living for years. This might are due to desperation in the past or because there was just nothing available to eat–being unwell or religion. Most belief systems have fasting times, proving that it's a doable, good, and generally a quite natural way.

Yes, there are many shreds of evidence to point out that 'starving' yourself a touch a day can have a really good impact on your health–not just your weight. This is often because it takes six to eight hours for your body to metabolize your glycogen stores, and then you begin to burn fat. Furthermore, if you replenish this glycogen by consuming only every 8 hours, the body would find it much harder to use your fat stores as food. Essentially, to encourage your body to do what must be done, you would like to make sure you give yourself an opportunity from the food.

What Is Obesity and What Causes It?

Obesity may be a complex disease that involves an unhealthy amount of body fat. It's a medical condition that increases the probabilities of getting other diseases and health problems, like a heart condition, diabetes, high vital sign, and certain cancers.

There is a spread of reasons why some people are having difficulty preventing obesity. Typically, obesity is that the results of a mixture of genetic causes, alongside the environment and private diet and exercise choices.

The good news is that even moderate weight loss will boost or avoid obesity-related health problems. Dietary changes increased physical activity, and behavioral changes will assist you in reducing. Prescription medications and weightless treatments are potential choices for the treatment of obesity.

What Causes Obesity?

Obesity is often complex. You gain weight because you eat more calories than you're employed out. Yet the load could also be suffering from certain variables. They include;

- **What and the way you eat:** In today's culture, consuming unhealthy foods and over-eating is straightforward? Many things, including emotions, habits, and access to food, can influence eating behavior.

- **How active are you?** New conveniences— like elevators, vehicles, and tv remote control— attempt to avoid such conveniences. Being active helps you stay fit and healthy. You burn more calories when you're fit, albeit you're sleeping.

- **Your genetic makeup:** The impact of your genetic makeup on your weight is extremely high. It affects;

    o The rate at which the body uses energy (calories) in rest is named the basal rate. Many of us are born with higher metabolic baseline levels than others. They burn more calories, of course than others.

    o You can increase your rate through regular physical activity.

    o Low-calorie foods are getting to lower the rate. If you do not burn calories as quickly, a high rate makes it easier to realize weight.

    o Signals from your body, like your hunger, feeling hungry or full.

    o Distribution of your fat. You've got no control over how your body stores fat. Women hold more fat in the hips and thighs. When women age, the belly accumulates more fat.

- **A diet high in carbohydrates**. It's not clear what role carbohydrates play in weight gain. Carbohydrates increase blood sugar levels, which in effect induce pancreatic insulin release, and insulin stimulates fat tissue production and may cause weight gain. Most scientists believe that straightforward carbohydrates (sugars, fructose, desserts, soft drinks, alcohol, wine, etc.) contribute to weight gain because they're ingested more easily into the bloodstream than complex carbohydrates (pasta, rice, beans, potatoes, fresh fruits, etc.) and thus induce a more noticeable release of insulin in meals than complex carbohydrates. Some scientists believe that this higher release of insulin results in weight gain.

- **Feeding frequency**. There's some debate about the connection between feeding frequency (how often you eat) and weight. There are many studies that overweight people eat less often than normal-weight people. Scientists have observed that folks who eat small meals four or five times each day have lower levels of cholesterol and lower and/or more healthy levels of blood glucose than people that eat less often (two or three large meals a day). One possible explanation is that tiny, regular meals yield steady levels of insulin, whereas large meals after meals cause large spikes in insulin.

- **Psychological factors**. Emotions impair eating habits for a few individuals. In reaction to feel like depression, sorrow, pain, or frustration, often people eat excessively. While most overweight people haven't any more health symptoms than normal-weight people, binge eating is problematic for about 30% of individuals seeking look after serious weight issues.

- **Disease**. Those associated with obesity are conditions like hypothyroidism, insulin resistance, polycystic ovary syndrome, and Cushing's syndrome. Many disorders can cause obesity, like Prader-Willi syndrome.

8. Social issues: social issues are linked to obesity. Lack of cash to get healthy food or lack of safe walking or fitness facilities will increase the danger of obesity.

A Word About Metabolism

The way we lose or gain weight is primarily thanks to our metabolism. Simply put, these are the chemicals that turn food into energy inside our bodies. to make this process possible, we'd like four primary macronutrients:

- Proteins
- Fats
- Carbohydrates

- Nucleic acids (present in DNA)

Then our bodies break down and use the items we consume for energy. The pace at which this is often done determines what proportion of weight we gain or lose. A broad number of things influence this pace, including:

- Age–the older you become, the slower the metabolism becomes.
- Body size–your body will need to work much harder to urge the work done if you're larger or heavier.
- Muscle mass–higher muscle mass also leads to a metabolism that's more efficient.
- Sex–males are metabolized more easily than women.
- Level of activity–workout features a huge impact on how the metabolism functions. The more you progress, the higher.
- Hormonal causes–you are going to be suffering from certain hormones and related diseases.
- Genetics–you should be ready to see how your body functions from the history of your family.
- Environmental factors–the rate could also be influenced by the environment. If it's extremely hot or cold, for this process to figure, your body must work even harder.
- Diet–healthy eating can only help your body work more efficiently when you're tired and on time.

- Medicines–prescription medicines, caffeine, and nicotine can hamper your metabolism.

As you'll see from this list, the sole belongings you can control over from this list are muscle mass and exercise— you'll work to enhance this — and diet and drugs— what you've decided to place in your body can decide how it functions and behaves. Fasting is extremely useful to hurry up your metabolism, as shown by the subsequent points:

- This removes waste from the body produced from regular eating and drinking. This may provide a boost to your metabolism.
- Activates the human somatotropin that creates the body burn fat to stay the muscle working.
- This controls digestion, promoting healthy bowel activity, and helping to enhance the rate.
- This controls blood glucose, so you do not get ravenous (which people often desire they go to).
- This improves your eating habits as you would like to make the foremost of your calorie limit. Healthy eating provides the best chance for your metabolism to function at its maximum pace.
- Fasting slows down the aging process, helping to stay the metabolism healthier for an extended .

Calorie restriction will help us shed weight and feel far better, as you've got seen, but this is often extremely challenging because appetite is one among our key drivers. Research has shown, luckily, that intermittent fasting may be a much safer thanks to achieving an equivalent result.

What Happens Once You Eat

Protein, fats, and starch are the most components of food. Protein is significant to the body's internal and cellular repair; protein is employed in the cells for development and nutrition through excess fat accumulation, while carbohydrates are energy given foods. Carbohydrates are converted into glucose for energy in the bloodstream, and this is often commonly mentioned as "blood sugar." If sugar becomes excess in the system, it becomes toxic; thus, the pancreas releases insulin that brings the surplus glucose into the liver and muscles to be processed as glycogen. Many of the foods we eat can increase the event of insulin, and therefore the remaining insulin starts to create up over an extended period of your time, allowing the body to create insulin resistance. There's weight gain at this stage, which contributes to obesity.

An average person will store up to fifteen grams of glycogen weight per pound. The leftovers are processed as fat when there's excess glycogen in the blood. With the disorganized and disproportionate way people eat nowadays, the body waits around for glucose from foods, which it then stores as fat for a fasting period that never comes. This results in an imbalance in energy levels because carbohydrate is being consumed regularly instead of using the fat that has been stored in the body. Such lifestyle results in weight gain, obesity, and diabetes.

What Happens Once You Fast

Rather than use glucose when the body is fasting, it switches to fatty acids. This process happens when there's a rise in lipolysis (the breakdown of stored fat in your white fat into fatty acids and glycerol in the bloodstream). The free fatty acids are then used for energy, repair, and growth. In the event they're not used, they're re-esterified as fat in your body.

The fatty acids in the bloodstream start to extend 12 hours after your last meal. This suggests that each one body fat starts to float around in the blood, waiting to be used. In 24 hours of fasting, the quantity of fatty acids reduces drastically in 72 hours, the fatty acids peak and plateau. When fasting, the body releases twice the quantity of fat into the bloodstream that's needed for the traditional body function. People are always scared that they will not have the specified energy to hold out their daily duties, but fasting actually makes the body oversaturated with fatty acids, which makes the body have an excess amount of energy. Muscles and other tissues increase their ability to store fat when fasting; therefore, extra fatty acids could also be stored there or utilized in different biosynthetic and metabolic pathways.

Fasting encourages the organs in the body to use and store fat. When fasting, the fat in the body does not sit as a backup energy source; instead, it's getting used by the body. this manner of burning fat is named "fat-burning mode." In this era, the body becomes super-efficient at processing fat, which suggests tissues and other organs in the body use the fat for energy.

The Body's Reaction To Fasting

Here's what's happening to your body in a fasting period:

- **Body fat breakdown:** This is the part that contributes to weight loss and helps to scale back the danger of heart condition, strokes, obesity, diabetes, etc.
- **Cholesterol deposits break down:** Waste is removed easily through a fast—and this involves cholesterol, which is typically contained inside the vessel lining. The cholesterol levels may very well rise because the body detoxifies in the primary week of the fast, but it'll decrease.
- **Mechanical fibrinolysis:** Dangerous blood clots are often weakened more easily while you're on a quick. This method is mentioned as fibrinolysis.
- **Speeding up autolysis:** Every cell in the body has its own destruction's seeds. If the necessity emerges, the cell can

release and self-destruct its own self-destructive enzymes. It's autolysis. At the pace, the autolysis process results in the breakdown of this sort of tissue that has inhibited normal functioning.

- **Lower diuresis:** Diuresis is that the elimination of salt and water from the kidneys. The body naturally and automatically removes salt and water while fasting without destroying the tissues of the body. This diuresis may be a tremendous benefit to wellbeing.

- **The phagocytosis has intensified:** When fasting, the body's protective army of white blood cells is increasing its ability to destroy virulent bacteria and digest waste. The fasting person's white blood cells were far more effective in killing virulent bacteria.

Fundamentals of Intermittent Fasting

Intermittent fasting may be a food consumption methodology that alternates between the limitation of calorie consumption or skipping meals and, therefore, the usual food consumption in a particular period of time. There are various sorts of intermittent fasting routines, like the 5:2 diet, and lots of more. The foremost famous sort of intermittent fasting is that the 16:8 method, which comprises eating in an 8-hour timeframe before skipping meals for 16 hours.

Weight loss is the commonest factor for people to aim intermittent fasting. By allowing you to consume fewer meals, intermittent fasting may result in an instantaneous decrease in calorie intake.

Furthermore, intermittent fasting alters hormone levels to assist in losing weight. Additionally, to lessening insulin levels and elevating human somatotropin (HGH) levels, it increases the expulsion of the fat reduction hormone. Due to these alterations in hormones, temporary fasting may elevate your rate by a maximum of 14%. As a result of you consuming less and reducing your calorie intake, intermittent fasting causes weight reduction by altering both parts of the calorie equation.

Researchers have found that intermittent fasting is often a robust weight reduction tool. It's known that this consuming pattern may result in a 3 to eight percent weight loss over 1 to six months, which may be a huge amount if compared to tons of weight reduction research. Individuals who reduced 4 to 7 percent of their waistline also showed an enormous reduction of dangerous belly fat that accumulates around your organs and leads to illnesses.

Intermittent fasting causes less muscle loss than the more conventional technique of general limiting of one's calorie intake. However, it's important to take into consideration that the first factor for its triumph is that intermittent fasting encourages you to consume fewer calories. If you consume massive amounts of food once you do eat, you'll not lose any weight in the least.

Intermittent fasting is primarily utilized as a weight reduction routine. But it's proven it's going to even be advantageous to one's health in various ways.

For instance, intermittent fasting has been shown to reduce inflammation and enhance brain responsiveness and glucose levels. This is often why intermittent fasting is an eating pattern that comprises cycling between the stages in which you normally eat or skip meals.

Skipping Meals

When you skip meals, tons of things can occur in your body, particularly on the extent of hormones and cells. For instance, your body calibrates hormone levels to permit quick access to your storage of body fat. Your cells also start crucial fixing processes and alter the structure of genes.

Here are some alterations that happen in your body once you skip meals:

- **Human Growth Hormone (HGH)**: The human growth hormone significantly increases, rising to a minimum of 5 times quite the quality amount. This is often beneficial for losing weight and gaining muscle mass.
- **Insulin**: Sensitivity to insulin enhances, and insulin levels decrease significantly. Decreasing insulin levels transform body fat storage to make it accessible.
- **Cellular Repair**: once you skip meals, your cells start cellular fixing processes. This includes autophagy, where cells absorb good proteins and expel bad proteins that accumulate inside cells.
- **Gene Expression**: There are alterations in the usage of genes linked to long lifespan and security against disease.

These alterations in hormone levels, cell usage, and gene characteristics are a number of the most health advantages of intermittent fasting. Once you skip meals, HGH levels rise, and insulin levels decrease. Your body's cells alter the characteristics of genes and begin crucial cellular fixation processes.

Aging and Intermittent Fasting

People are trying to find the key to remaining young, healthy, and fit centuries. The worldwide anti-aging market contributed to US$ 42.51 billion in 2018 and is predicted to cross US$ 55 billion by 2023. nobody has discovered the elusive cure to debar depression, weight gain, joint pain, and every one the opposite, not so fun side effects of getting older, despite tons of cash funneling into science and rising consumer spending.

In addition to potential positive effects on the brain, intermittent fasting has well-documented age-related advantages. There are several ways in which prolonged fasting helps to hamper the aging process. The primary is minimal inflammation. Evidence has shown that IF is related to reduced brain inflammation, and therefore the effect in other tissues has been seen by other studies.

Inflammation may be a biological defense mechanism that happens naturally when threats like a compromised enzyme, poisonous agent, or pathogen are identified by the system. However, if inflammation kicks up too often or gets out of control, it can cause chronic body-wide inflammation, resulting in tissue damage or illness. A summary of how inflammation is caused and addressed in a 2016 literature review found that an excessive amount of can cause disorder, atherosclerosis, type 2 diabetes, atrophic arthritis, and a few cancers. In short, keeping inflammation under check using IF can keep us healthy for an extended .

According to the study, the second process by which IF tends to delay aging is by reducing the aggregation of molecules weakened by free radicals. Free radicals are toxic compounds capable of destroying cells, causing aging and disease.

Health Benefits of Intermittent Fasting for Women

There is a general belief that intermittent fasting is often detrimental to your health, which is completely wrong. These are a number of the health and lifestyle benefits that come from intermittent fasting.

- It increases your lifespan: studies have proven that one among the explanations for an extended lifetime is intermittent fasting. While the whole process is unknown, the anti-aging benefits of fasting may come from the increased insulin sensitivity and, therefore, the reduction of insulin and insulin-like peptides. Intermittent fasting alters the aging effects of genes by decreasing oxidative stress while strengthening immunity and energy metabolism.

- It makes the body immune to stress: almost like exercise, intermittent fasting may be a mild stressor to the body, which makes the cells immune to stress.

- Autophagy: In fasting, the body is forced to wash up by recycling old, damaged, and unused proteins. Autophagy is important for cells to survive because it discourages the buildup of poisons, which may cause frailty and atrophy while supporting muscle mass. Aging and anti-aging diseases are bogged down drastically by autophagy.

- It supports the system and increases disease resistance: Intermittent fasting is extremely beneficial to the system because it stops inflammatory responses, reduces oxidative damage, and increase stress resistance. Research has shown that intermittent fasting changes the organic phenomenon on a cellular level and regulating inflammatory responses. Intermittent fasting increases the power of the white blood cells to phagocytize (the process by which they breakdown and eliminate bacteria and other toxins). While fasting, the liver stores less fat, and this makes it resistant to insulin resistance, which prevents liver diseases like non-alcoholic liver disease. The resistance benefits reach the brain and protect it against neurodegenerative diseases like Alzheimer's, Parkinson, Huntington's diseases, and stroke.

- It prevents against cancer: Intermittent fasting reduces the danger of cancer and cell proliferation drastically. It works effectively on certain cancerous cells and protects them from oxidative stress while stopping the expansion of cancerous cells without protecting them from oxidative stress.

- It increases insulin sensitivity: Intermittent fasting reduces fasting insulin and prevents insulin resistance and, therefore, the various problems which may develop, like metabolic syndrome, obesity, and diabetes. Other benefits of increased insulin sensitivity are nutrition partitioning, decreased appetite, weight loss, and lowered cholesterol.

- It encourages the expansion of the human growth hormone: Contrary to popular belief that intermittent fasting causes stunted growth, it actually promotes the expansion of the human somatotropin (HGH). HGH stimulates cell reproduction and regeneration. As we get older, the assembly of HGH reduces. Since consuming food blocks the HGH release, intermittent fasting acts as a double negative in removing the stoppers of HGH. The increased secretion of HGH increases lipolysis and fat burning.

- It enhances brain function: In intermittent fasting, the central system will receive a continuing stream of fatty acids and ketones, which can make your brain alert and active. Ketones are good for learning and memory, and it also slows the nervous disorder processes. The brain functions better with ketones instead of glucose. Intermittent fasting increases your alertness by increasing norepinephrine, a neurotransmitter that increases concentration. Intermittent fasting helps the brain with anti-aging and protects it from oxidative and metabolic stress. It aids in the production of neurogenesis, also as neuroplasticity. Intermittent fasting increases "brain-derived neurotrophic factor," which helps the brain neurons in resisting dysfunction and regeneration.

- It elevates the mood: Meal patterns play a big influence on how you are feeling. Intermittent fasting encourages an honest mood by increasing the discharge of norepinephrine and dopamine levels. Intermittent fasting controls the blood glucose levels and insulin, which stops the sensation of being angry when your blood glucose drops. A study conducted in 2014 on non-diabetic adults showed fluctuating sugar levels were related to anger, and high levels of blood glucose made it difficult to regulate anger.

10. It enhances your exercise life: Intermitted fasting helps maximize fat oxidation, increases muscular oxidative capacity, and prevents low levels of blood glucose. Intermittent fasting also the synthesis of muscle protein.

Side Effects of Fasting

Intermittent fasting is often detrimental to your health if you're affected by medical conditions that involve the guts and liver. However, there are medical conditions that will cause stomach discomfort on an empty stomach like NSAIDs, ASAs, iron supplements, and metformin, which makes it imperative that you simply consult your doctor on the way to combine your daily medications. In the event you are feeling dizzy or ill, it's recommended that you simply stop your fasting immediately. Always monitor your blood work and vital sign regularly. You would possibly get to adjust your medications to avoid hypoglycemia, which may be life-threatening. In the event you cannot monitor yourself, or there's no doctor accessible, it's advisable that you simply don't last for long periods.

Common Misconceptions About Intermittent Fasting

There are tons of misconceptions when it involves intermittent fasting, and it's imperative to clarify these myths.

- Intermittent fasting slows down metabolic rates: Studies have shown that frequent meals boost metabolism; while this is often true, it's also important to notice that intermittent fasting also does an equivalent. Research has shown that intermittent fasting increases the body metabolism by 3.6-14%; although other factors can determine whether you reduce.

- Intermittent fasting causes muscle loss: Muscle loss can only happen when intermittent fasting is completed wrongly; when done correctly, you will not be losing muscle as long as you're eating enough protein. When eating, confirm it's a diet and also combine it with resistance training. You will not lose muscles or atrophy because you're burning the glycogen stored in the muscle.

- Fasting lowers your testosterone levels: this is often a touch more complicated because research has shown that prolonged fasting reduces the testosterone levels, but it increases to a better level after weeks of fasting. With shorter fasting periods (24 hours), the testosterone levels increase exponentially. Research has shown that testosterone increases exponentially 20-30 more in fasting than when in a fed state. The rationale behind the increase in testosterone is because fasting may be a sort of stress on the body. Stress stimulates cortisol levels, which cause the assembly of testosterone also as somatotropin elevation, which maintains muscle mass.

- The brain needs a daily supply of dietary glucose to function: there's a belief that if you do not eat carbs every few hours, your brain will pack up because the brain uses glucose for fuel. This is often entirely untrue because the body produces glucose through a process called gluconeogenesis. In prolonged fasting or very low carbs diets, the body produces ketone from dietary fats. Ketone is a replacement for glucose, and this makes the brain less hooked into glucose.

- Easting regularly is sweet for your health: Short term fasting helps the body to repair old and dysfunctional cells, and this process is named autophagy. Autophagy helps to guard against diseases like cancer, aging, and Alzheimer's disease. Research has shown that regular snacking is detrimental to your health and increases your chance of diseases. Studies have shown that foods that contain high calories increase your chance of liver fat, and other people who eat more have a better risk of colorectal cancer.

- Intermittent fasting is harmful to your health: you would possibly have heard that intermittent fasting is dangerous for your health, but studies have shown that that's quite the reverse. It's been proven that it changes your organic phenomenon, which is liable for longevity and immunity. It's also beneficial for metabolic health, insulin sensitivity; it reduces oxidative stress, inflammation, and a heart condition. It boosts brain health by increasing the amount of brain-derived neurotrophic factor (BDNF), a hormone that protects against depression and other psychological state conditions.

- Intermittent fasting may be a sort of starvation diet: If you skip a meal for 24-48 hours, you will not starve. Studies have shown that you simply need to fast for quite 60 hours straight before your resting rate drops.

Starvation is suffering or death caused by hunger. In starvation, the fat stores in the body are depleted, and your body must breakdown muscle tissue for energy. In intermittent fasting, the body releases the fat, and therefore the muscle and lean tissue are untouched. Unless it's a particularly prolonged fast and your fat levels are below 4%, intermittent fasting won't affect any muscle or lean tissue as long because it is correctly through with the assistance of a dietitian or physician.

- Once you aren't fasting, you'll eat whatever you like: it's important to notice that you simply won't reduce once you fast if you exceed the number of calories you consume on your off days. It's advisable to eat a diet that has fruits, vegetables, and whole grains. If you're not under any dietary restrictions, you'll try fish, lean meat, eggs, beans, poultry, and nuts.

- Intermittent fasting is bad for women: this is often an issue that's commonly asked from women, and there are conflicting reports from experts. Premenopausal women may experience changes in their hormones in intermittent fasting, but this only happens when there's a protracted fast. It'd not be easy for a few women to undergo intermittent fasting because they're more vulnerable to stress.

Some women fast for 20 hours straight a day, and that they don't experience hormonal changes. This is often mainly hooked into the genetic makeup of the lady as some can adapt well to worry that's related to intermittent fasting, while others cannot bear it. It's advisable to start out small and gradually increase the periods of intermittent fasting in order that your body can slowly adapt to the changes.

- Gorge and assume you'll still lose some fat: Intermittent fasting is extremely effective when it involves fat loss. Regular checks aren't needed; all you would like to do is stop eating processed foods and stick with regular wholesome foods.

The Common Lies Of Weight Loss

- **The less you weigh, the healthier you're**

You are not defined by the amount on the size, nor does it represent how safe you're. The goal of a journey of weight loss should be quite just working to bring down the amount on the size. Once you eat healthily and exercise regularly, thanks to a rise in muscle mass, you'll even feel a little touch bit of weight gain. Muscle is denser than fat, consistent with studies, and takes up less space in the body. It means you'll shed fat and gain muscle, but while keeping an equivalent weight, look leaner.

- **You ought to only eat 1,200 calories each day**

Although counting calories when trying to reduce is significant, it doesn't suggest you'll limit yourself to the 1,200 calories that are often called the magic amount. The rate of every person is different, which means the amount at which calories are consumed by our bodies is additionally different. Research says those with more muscle appear to possess metabolism above those with more body fat. And since the makeup of the body varies from individual to individual, every one is exclusive in the number of calories we burn all day long. It ensures that there's no fixed number of calories that everybody should be shooting for.

- **You ought to cut out certain food groups**

Carbohydrates are one of the foremost important nutrients that our bodies got to function. Research notes that they supply energy to the body, can help reduce the danger of the disorder , and are required for weight control. In many various foods, including fruits and vegetables, carbohydrates are included. So, it isn't practical to settle on to urgently obviate carbohydrates completely and reduce. Have the odd slice of pizza and piece of cake to satisfy cravings, but don't completely stop major food groups as you would like to reduce. The likelihood is that you are going to limit yourself an excessive amount of, which can encourage you to eat an excessive amount of later.

- **Following a particular diet trend will assist you in reducing**

There are numerous different diet patterns, from diets and veganism that are gluten-free. The truth is, eating vegan exclusively or unexpectedly cutting gluten won't allow you to lose 10 pounds instantly. Dieting has many health benefits, but unless you find out how to raised nourish your body after these habits, you'll gain weight rather than losing it. Confirm you recognize where you'll get your carbohydrates, fats, and protein from before you adopt any new eating plan.

- **Weight-loss supplements will cause you to be skinny**

The trick to weight loss isn't to drink diet teas and take fat-burning supplements. Many scientists say little or no research has been done to point out how effective weight-loss pills are often, so it's impractical to rely entirely on them to urge in shape. You ought to follow a healthy diet and exercise regularly rather than counting on fat-burning pills or detox teas. Anything that promises an answer that's quick and straightforward is perhaps just a scam.

Facts About Intermittent Fasting

Here are some details that you simply might not realize intermittent fasting, but should be before you continue.

- **Methods in intermittent fasting are supported years of research**

Animal fasting study dates back to eighty years. Reports on human fasting are dating back a minimum of six years. More and more clinical trials are being administered.

- **'Starvation mode' may be a myth**

In the 1950s, the study suggesting starvation had negative effects was administered. They took a bunch of young men in this research and told them to survive on about half their usual calories and that they tracked them for six months, obviously losing drastic amounts of weight. And when their body fat fell to 5 pounds, they began experiencing major problems. Now that's a very, really extremely easy for a very while, this experiment didn't have an honest foundation, and therefore the weight loss was made far timely. It obviously led to negative health issues. Intermittent fasting is not any such thing.

- **Medical research also begins with self-experimentation**

Before you are doing it, you'll not skills quickly; it can work for you. Most are special, most are peculiar, and it is vital to always bear in mind. Maybe not for you, what does for others. If you do not like one easily, try another.

- **Fasting sporadic causes, you to shed weight, not muscle**

A standard diet will cause you to lose around 75% fat, 25% muscle. It's between 85 and one hundred pc fat for intermittent fasting.

- **Not all fasts are made equal: intermittent fasting is not any juice fasting**

To ensure that you simply include all food groups, remember what you eat in a quick. A glass of juice may be a sugar hit. Which will cause you to feel hungry, and it'll make the amount of insulin go up.

- **Dementia may be a nutrition problem**

The impact of food isn't just physical. It can have mental effects too. It's going to even have mental effects. Keep this in mind when considering the straightforward intermittent and, therefore, the food you dine in it.

- **'The fast diet' remains a piece ongoing**

Tests on intermittent fasting are still to be done. Another thing that has been known is that it's much easier for people to stay than other diets. The foremost effective thanks to losing fat and hold off the load have been noticed by many test subjects.

- **Nothing must hold you back**

You may worry about your age, health condition, or something like that, but as long as you ask a health care professional before you go—to get some personalized advice—you are often confident you're doing it in a healthy way.

Getting Started with Intermittent Fasting

Determine Your Goals

As crucial as incorporating the fast into your lifestyle is, it's vital that you simply care about what you would like to urge out of the fast also. If you're unhappy with the results, it's doubtful you'll proceed with the lifestyle change you've initiated – all of your energy is going to be wasted.

When watching your goals, it's always advisable to use the SMART acronym:

- Specific
- Measurable
- Attainable
- Realistic
- Time-bound.

An example of making a sensible goal for your fast would work like this:

- **Specific** – It must be made more specific. I'm getting to lose 10 pounds.'

- **Measurable** – How will you create sure you retain up with this? I will be able to quickly follow the 5 2 – pick Monday and Thursday as my fast days.'

- **Attainable** – can this be done? Will it always be appropriate on Mondays and Thursdays? If you do not have a backup plan. Wednesday goes to be my day of backup.

- **Realistic**–Will you actually be ready to stick with the calories of 500/600 on the two fast days? Would you eat healthily in the meantime? If you're uncertain, you ought to seek advice from your doctor before you proceed. I'm getting to test myself with a quick 24-hour first.'

- **Time-bound** – you are going to take to stay an eye fixed on your growth; you're heading to your target. I'm getting to weigh myself hebdomadally .'

Making targets in this manner has been shown to possess advantages and can assist you in achieving them. They're far more organized, they're clearly possible, and that they don't have anything to carry you back. Print this data and reserve it for you to use a day in a convenient location. Make yourself accountable.

Select the Best Time to Start

Once you've found out which program you would like to follow, you will need to work out the foremost suitable hours for yourself to abstain from eating. You're likely to take to incorporate the hours you're spending in the easy—so it is a bit easier. You will have to work out the remainder of it around your lifestyle and job.

Most fasts have a dictation about what percentage meals or treats you need to eat every day. Others are more complex, leaving you with the choice. So, are you getting to have one or two meals or five or six snacks? Thanks to the limited time and therefore, the way we usually work, most of the people prefer to have up to three meals each day. Another approach is additionally simpler because it allows the body the capability to digest food more efficiently.

Choose Foods to Incorporate

One of the foremost commonly asked fasting questions is, 'what am I able to eat?' Most diets don't say, but on the non-fasting days, it is often hard to understand what 'eat as usual' entails. It also can be a struggle on your fasting days to urge the foremost out of your approved calories. You continue to want to urge all you would like to be ready to work rightly.

Prepare Yourself

One of the foremost difficult things to coach for a quick is getting past your food addiction. this might be something you do not even know you've, but below may be a list of signs to seem for:

- Once you begin eating certain foods, you finish up eating quite expected.
- Although you're not hungry, you retain certain eating foods.
- You're eating to the purpose of feeling sick.
- You're concerned about not eating certain food types or about lowering on certain food types.
- You leave you thanks for getting them when other things aren't available.
- You eat certain foods so often or in such large quantities that you simply start eating food instead of studying, spending time together with your family, or doing recreational activities.
- You avoid occupational or social environments in which certain foods are available, thanks to fear of excessive consumption.
- Due to food and eating, you've got problems working well at your job or college.

If this is often the case, you'll get to get some help from a health care provider. This condition is often troublesome and should compete together with your dieting. It's usually related to food, but also can be related to carbs, which can also cause problems together with your speed. Below are some tips to assist with this:

- Look at the matter, not the symptom–these addictions are often connected with something greater than simply food. It can assist you tons to repair this.
- Eliminate processed foods–this quite food is toxic, and getting obviate it'll only cause you to healthier.
- Be careful–it is going to be challenging, of course, but you've got to stay with it. The worst, but also the foremost rewarding, are going to be the primary 48 hours.
- Kill old habits–figure out once you eat badly and specialize at that moment.
- Increase the dosage slowly–don't roll in the hay timely because you are going to possess trouble.
- Follow your nutritional needs–whatever you are doing, confirm you get all you would like.
- Have a cheat meal–don't starve yourself or find it harder to heal.

Another area where planning is important while you fast is exercise. The diet will change, counting on the times you do not eat, and knowing which will benefit you at the end of the day.

It is mentioned that exercising on an empty stomach potentially features a lot of advantages – if this is often something you'd wish to know. These include:

- Decreased body fat
- Increased muscular tonus
- Improved aerobic agility and consistency
- Potential to satisfy your fitness goals much faster
- Improvement in strength and concupiscence
- Stronger skin and decreased wrinkles

It is advised that you simply do an interval training to urge the foremost out of your exercise. You ought to haven't any trouble eating while you fast as long as you schedule your meals accordingly. Here's a thought you'll do of an easy workout:

- Warm-up for 3 minutes.

 Walk for 30 seconds as hard and as fast as possible. You'll gasp for air and appearance, such as you won't be ready to continue another few seconds. It's better to use lower resistance and better repetitions to extend your pulse.

- Recover for 90 seconds, still going, but at a slower pace.
- Do the workout with high intensity and regeneration seven times more.

Remembering that fasting isn't almost weight loss is extremely important. It also can assist you in building muscle mass—as the various diets included in this article have shown. Here are some recommendations on the way to work out and build muscle as fast as you do:

- Late-night training sessions will assist you to manage your calories.
- In the recovery period, you'll include protein and carbohydrates in your meal.
- Use the bulk of your calories—approximately 60%—to help your body recover right following your exercise.
- Eat about 20 percent of your daily calories before you're employed bent offer you the strength you are going to wish (while it isn't really important as mentioned above, but should help build muscle mass).
- Do not exclude all fats—retain' healthy' fats as a serious part of your diet.
- Try to eat by 5 am—it is suggested to eat early instead of later.

When building muscle is not the ultimate goal, and fasting is more about burning fat, you would possibly also try mixing aerobic workouts like biking, surfing, and athletics with one among the fasting diets. For the simplest results, it's really advised to do a minimum of some exercise alongside your fasting. Not only will you see your efforts perform even easier, but earlier, you'll also begin to feel better and healthier. You're liberal to choose an honest exercise regime, as long as you are doing something.

Whatever the ultimate goal, remembering what you are doing after you're employed out is extremely important. This is often some time of recovery until your body gets up. This is often the foremost important time for weight loss and muscle building, so you would like to line up an excellent schedule to urge the foremost out of your exercise.

You should do the following:

- Cooldown—do some quite light exercise to encourage your body to relax and hamper your pulse. It's recommended to take five minutes.
- Stretch—you can stretch then. The muscles compress, and you are not getting to want them to shorten. This may help the body to recover rightly.
- Drink water—fill-up fluid levels. Drink 2 or 3 cups after you've done your workout for two hours.
- Refuel—after exercise, feeding is additionally necessary. It allows you to strengthen your muscles and increase your levels of energy. This must be done in 90 minutes of completing the exercise. Include in this meal or snack protein and carbohydrates.

Things to Remember

The whole time you're fasting, there are things to stay in mind, to stay you going. These include:

- One day at a time —don't worry about the longer-term an excessive amount of, just reflect on where you're.
- Goals—that is to mention, always confine mind your goals for inspiration.
- Caffeine—it's perfect for the pick-me-ups you'll like along the way.
- Water—stay hydrated. That's really important.
- Rewards—please reward yourself for realizing your goals. This may allow you to remain motivated. It needn't be nutritional rewards; you ought to search for it outside the box.
- Nutrition —consider other nutrition-free remedies. You ought to retrain the brain even as much so as to enjoy healthy snacks. It only takes a touch a little bit of time.
- Don't get trapped in the rules—it is often unhelpful to rely an excessive amount of on the' dos and don'ts.'
- Don't be too harsh on yourself—it's not the top of the planet, albeit you create mistakes. You'll continue again in the least times.

- Don't binge–don't get too wild once you can actually eat again. it'll cause you to feel horrible and can kill much of your diligence.
- Prepare–if you're committed to having something from all of your food groups, it's possible that your quick is going to be higher. You would possibly just got to prepare your meals before time.

Just Start

So, you're happy now! There's nothing holding you back once you've taken all of those moves, so get going. No more excuses, no more caution, just continue. The longer you set it off, the more likely you're never getting to start. So, don't say' I'm getting to start on Tuesday," I'm getting to roll in the hay on the primary day of the month,' or' I'm getting to start when that's done.' If there is no real reason you are going to urge in your way, just go!

Here are the sensible steps to recapped starting:

- Set your goal–pick your target and keep it in mind. Choose a fasting plan that supported your target and lifestyle. And confirm you stick with it, it's to be realistic. It'll never happen if it's just unlikely!
- Make your promise–make sure you stick with it once you set your mind to sporadic tempo. Do whatever it takes to make

sure you are not going off track–even if meaning telling someone and ensuring they hold you accountable.

- Prepare and plan–get it beat order. Confirm you are not holding anything back. Once the fasting is embedded in your daily routine, it'll be smoother, but the primary few days and weeks are going to be where the most important challenge lies. Confirm you'll relax as required, but you've got enough diversion to stay you going.

- Store–Make sure you've got in your cupboards all the food you are going to wish. You do not want to offer up those excuses. This also refers to facilities for workouts.

How to Fast Intermittently

There are alternative ways you'll fast, namely;

The 16:8 Method: Fast For 16 Hours A Day

This method includes fasting every day for 14-16 hours and limiting your "eating phase" to 8-10 hours. Inside the eating phase, you'll slot in 2, 3, or more meals. This strategy is additionally called the Lean gains routine. Following this approach to fasting are often equivalent to not having anything after your last meal and skipping breakfast subsequent day.

In the case that you simply finish your last eating phase at 8 p.m. and do not eat until 12 noon the subsequent day, at that specific time, you're already skipping eating for 16 hours between meals.

It is more advisable for ladies because it's 14-15 hours of fasting, which is best as they're more aware of short-paced fasting.

For those that are trying to reduce, it is often difficult to become acclimated to skipping breakfast from the outset since their body is presumably to crave breakfast upon awakening. However, several breakfast enthusiasts eat tremendously alongside said phase.

You can drink liquids (non-caloric) in the skipping meals phase, and this will help lessen hunger levels. It's mandatory to consume solid foods in your eating phase. This would possibly not work if you eat portions of non-nutritious foods or if you exceed your allowed measures of calories.

People can consider this a usual approach to intermittent fasting. I also believe it myself and find it completely easy to follow. I eat a low-carb diet, so my hunger is managed fairly well. I do not feel hungry until around 1 p.m. onwards. This is often why I eat my Last Supper around 6-9 p.m., so as a result, I fast for about 16-19 hours.

To conclude, the 16:8 strategy includes day to day fasts of 16 hours for men and 14-15 hours for ladies. Every day, you lessen your food consumption to an 8-10 hour "eating phase" where you'll slot in 2-3 or more healthy meals.

The 20:4 Method: Fast For 20 Hours A Day

The 20:4 approach may be quite intermittent fasting that's reliant upon a 20-hour fast, with a 4-hour eating window. For the foremost part, you'll consume food in whatever amount you would possibly want in the 4-hour gap; however, it's hard to digest an excessive number of calories in such a brief period of your time.

The 4-hour eating window usually happens in the dark but can occur in any part of the day that suits you. For instance, you'll eat two dinners somewhere in the span of two p.m. and 6 p.m., and fast for about 20 hours.

This would be appropriate for people that are certain about intermittent fasting, are occupied in the day because they work and do not have the prospect to consume foods, do not feel hungry in the day, or find that eating makes them less productive and drowsy. This system is often implemented for unique events, no matter whether you are taking off for dinner or getting to devour a tasty meal with loved ones.

Extended Fasts

These are usually not done on a day to day but intermittently. These variations of fasts are great for people who have already determined that they cannot specialize in a daily fast; however, they could want to feature it into their weekly, monthly, or yearly timetable.

If you already practice restraint eating, you would possibly consider extensive fasting in the time to upgrade your ketosis to the subsequent level.

The 5:2 Diet: Fast For Two Days Out Of Each Week

This routine comprises of consuming foods for five days of the week while lowering calories right down to 500-600 on two days of the week. This eating routine is understood because of the "Fast Eating Regimen" and was formulated by Michael Mosley. In the fasting phase, it's recommended that ladies consume at the most 500 calories and men 600 calories at the most.

Moreover, you'll eat rightly on all days with the exception of Mondays and Thursdays (for example), where you eat two low-calorie meals (250 calories for every meal for ladies, and 300 for men).

As doubters continuously mention, there's no medical proof for the 5:2 eating routine itself, yet there are tons of notable advantages of intermittent fasting.

So, the 5:2 eating routine includes eating 500-600 calories for two days of the week but consuming foods daily on the opposite five days.

Eat-Stop-Eat: Do A 24-Hour Quick Fast

This includes a 24-hour quick fast a couple of times hebdomadally. This manner of eating has been mainstream for several years in the fitness world. By fasting from one meal, most likely the primary meal of each day, to the last meal continuously, this adds up to a 24-hour fast.

If you finished the last meal by Monday at 7 p.m., and haven't eaten anything until the last meal the subsequent day at 7 p.m., at that specific time, you've done a whole 24-hour fast. You refrain from eating meals from the primary meal to the primary meal or the second meal to the second meal. The ultimate product is the same.

Non-caloric liquid drinks are often consumed in the fasting phase. If you're doing this to urge fitter and healthier, then it's important that you simply typically eat in the eating time frames. As in, eat an equivalent amount of foods as if you've got not been fasting.

The issue with this system is that a whole 24-hour quick fast is often difficult for a few people. The way you do not need to put everything on the road immediately is to start with 14-16 hours, and continuing from that time onward is ok.

It is proven that the initial a part of the fasting phase is simple; however, I noticed that whenever I used to be doing it, I became voraciously ravenous when eating. I expected to use genuine discipline so as to finish the complete 24hours because a scarcity of control when it involves food consumption might end in failure.

To conclude, this routine is an intermittent fasting program that needs you to perform a couple of 24-hour fasts hebdomadally.

36-Hour Fasting

This is a singular sort of the 24-hour fast. You'll need to consume foods at the very beginning, fast for the sum of day two, and have breakfast on day three. This type of fasting can assist in your transition into ketosis or push you into a far better scenario of ketosis. This could be possible to do occasionally or as frequently as once every seven days, thirty days, or more.

The 42 Hour Fasting

This is 36 hours fast plus extra meal skip. In this system, you'll fast for a minimum of three days of the week and skip breakfast even in the non-fasting day.

The 72 Hour Protocol

This is commonly not considered a kind of intermittent fasting, but, ideally, you'll roll in the hay once a month or a minimum of 3 times a year. This fast helps to reboot the system through steam-based regeneration. It helps to stop cancer and other diseases. It helps in reducing the side effects of chemotherapy.

The Daily Meal-Based Fast

In this fasting approach, you eat a particular meal at different times of the day. For instance, you'll plan to eat breakfast and lunch while you skip dinner, lunch, and dinner while you skip breakfast or only dinner. With this sort of eating, you've got all the kinds of nutrients and calories for the day.

Alternate Day Fasting: Fast Every Other Day

This kind of fasting encourages you to skip meals every other day, but there are a couple of unique adaptations of this. A number of those routines allow the intake of roughly 500 calories in the fasting phase. Many consider that alternate day fasting demonstrates the medical advantages of intermittent fasting when utilized rightly. A full fast that's done every other day isn't for the faint-hearted because it's too hardcore, so I might not recommend this to individuals who are just trying to start out intermittent fasting.

With this routine, you'll be getting to roll in the hay the sensation of hunger a couple of times hebdomadally, which isn't desirable and advisable for the long-term. This approach involves skipping meals every other day, either by not eating anything or simply eating a couple of calories.

Unconstrained Fasting

This is one approach that I might recommend for a person who is hesitant about intermittent fasting or feels overpowered by going into unadvisable fasting times.

This is a fragile approach to intermittent fasting, which is driven by your way of life and body. It's perfect for people that prefer not to feel limited or get incapacitated if they do not meet the standards of their food consumption routine.

With this approach, you skip meals if you do not feel hungry or are too busy to recollect eating. Cooking and food consumption takes up tons of your time. Grasping the explanations why you eat will offer you the advantage to take different steps, like combining dinner with some recreational activities that also are beneficial for your health, like brisk walking or yoga. Mind conditioning may be a successful method to recondition the prevalent view that we've to eat three full meals per day.

Top Intermittent Fasting Protocols

Now that you are a bit more conversant in intermittent fasting – including explanations – it is time to delve into guidelines to assist you to opt which intermittent fast is best for you.

Three Day Fast

This pace is often achieved as often as possible. Most of the people who start a fasting plan to start with this, ascertain how they get on with it. At this point, however, you eat zero calories–drinking water only, so if three days look a touch daunting, you'll minimize it to 24 or 48 hours.

Best For: Beginners–those who want to ascertain how easily their body can cope.

How it works: at this point, you're just getting to drink water. There's no got to eat solid foods or other liquids. Attempt to drink one and a half to three liters of water in one day–a minimum of zero calories. If you affect any side effects, you'll get to pick a time to do this. The worst time to undertake this diet would be an excessively busy period fraught with pressures and deadlines–particularly for the very first time.

Pros: you are going to clear up your system and provides a way needed rest to your gastrointestinal system. In this point period, you'll also experience weight loss.

Cons: you've got some unpleasant side effects such as as-dizziness, nausea, etc. you'll also suffer hunger strikes, but by drinking a couple of glasses of water, you'll overcome that.

This can be an incredible thanks to starting by moving harder with less effort, in a quicker sprint—so you are going to start out learning how the body reacts before taking any longer decisions. It is often prudent to urge advice from a health care provider before you begin fast, particularly if it is your first, so you'll get some personalized advice that matches your case.

Eat Stop Eat

Best For happy eaters in need of an additional boost.

How It Works: Moderation is vital to the present fast. You'll still eat what you would like, but not such a lot. The fasting time is twice every week for twenty-four hours. At this point, no calories are eaten; on the other hand, you'll start eating as was common.

Here's an example of what proportion calories Brad Pilon—the diet founder—recommends you'll consume on a weekly basis, breaking the fast into two pieces (which some might find a far better thanks to doing it):

- Monday —eat 900 calories and begin fasting
- Tuesday—finish fasting and eat 1400 calories
- Wednesday—eat 1800 calories

- Thursday–eat 1800 calories
- Friday–eat 900 calories.
- Saturday – End fasting and eat 1200 calories
- Sunday – Eat 1800 calories

Of course, you would possibly eat a chocolate bar–but that's getting to take up an enormous chunk of your daily limit. It'll be nice to urge familiar with a calorie counter tool, like Calorie Counter, until you get won't to calculating your daily amount for yourself.

Pros: While 24 hours could seem sort of a while without food, the great news is that there's consistency in this plan. At the start, you do not need to go all or nothing. Go as long as you'll to assist your body to adapt the primary day without food and gradually increase the fasting process over time.

Cons: At the outset, this is often very likely to be a war. Symptoms like headache, exhaustion, or feeling cranky or anxious can occur. You'll also need a degree of self-control to make sure that after the fast, you do not binge directly.

This diet would cause you to believe what you set in your body, making it extremely healthy for your health. Once you start to concentrate on a more diet, you tend to reap the advantages. Here are some samples of what you'll get by eating a balanced diet:

- Regulating your weight—maintaining a healthy weight carries many other advantages with it. You are going to seem and feel tons better.

- The outlook will change, and you'll not only have better self-esteem, but it'll also even have positive mental consequences if you are feeling better about yourself.

- Eating right helps to regulate the vital sign, cholesterol, and blood flow. You'll lower the danger of heart condition, a stroke, and certain sorts of cancer to call only a couple of.

- Boosts your energy levels—if you've got less of that lethargic feeling, you'll be ready to do far more in a day. You're always getting to sleep better and feel far more rested.

- Improves health—living well will offer you a way greater opportunity to measure length.

The Warrior Diet

The Warrior Diet may be a higher eating level for the experienced faster. Do that as long as you recognize exactly how your body will react to long periods of failure to feed.

Best for: people that wish to follow the principles. This is often far better for those that need structure to navigate.

How it works: you are going to fast for 20 hours each day with this diet, eating an enormous meal in the dark. What you eat is important to its effectiveness in this fast. You ought to eat raw vegetables and fruit, fresh juice, and a couple of protein servings if desired in the fasting period. It's more about under-eating, instead of not eating in the least.

Thinking about what you are going to eat with this meal is additionally relevant. Whenever you eat raw food throughout the day, you'll be wanting to make certain that your meal includes protein, carbohydrates, and milk.

Pros: the power to snack can make it easier to urge through in the fasting period.

Cons: there are strict guidelines for what you eat, which will make it hard to maintain–especially when socializing.

You'll probably get to do this diet before you agree thereon. It is a big commitment to eat just one main meal each day. The advantage of doing this successfully, however, is often enormous:

- It boosts your metabolism.
- You see the general health change–from vitality to virility.
- Increase your lean muscle mass.
- The ageing process has been shown to hamper

Fat Loss Forever

This plan takes the simplest bits of the three above-mentioned plans. It's built to combine the fasting hours with satisfying individual needs–which means it's perfect because it can work for you. It boasts that for people that work long shifts, it's ideal because it's so adaptable to the requirements of anyone.

Best for: people that need flexibility in their fasting protocols.

How it works: you are going to fast with this program a day for varying amounts of hours. You're also getting to get one free day, followed by a quick of 36 hours.

Pros: you'll work into your crazy, busy lifestyle the varied fasting hours. This diet was designed to suit you, showing that everyone can do intermittent fasting.

Cons: you are going to possess to buy this package as it's tailored to you. Here may be a preview of 1 of the' 500 calorie' days to offer you a thought of what your diet could look like:

- Vegetables–1 serving, two times each day
- Fruit–1 serving, two times each day
- 100gm lean meat, two times each day
- 2 Thin Sunrice Rice Cakes or two melba toasts or two breadsticks–daily
- Juice of 1 lemon every day (optional)
- New herbs and spices–limitless for intermittent fasting.

Up-Day-Down-Day Diet

This diet's philosophy behind it's clear. One day, eat little or no, then eat the subsequent day as normal. Sometimes it's often mentioned as an alternate fasting day.

Best for: common weight-controlled goal dieters. At first, this may be a struggle, but in a study conducted by Dr Varaday, it had been observed that after only ten days, people found it easier to adopt the diet.

How it works: this diet is about eating normally at some point, as stated earlier, and consuming a limited amount of calories subsequent day. You'll eat 1 / 4 of your normal intake on the low-calorie days. Therefore 2,000 calories are going to be 400, and 500 are going to be 2,500 calories. Meal replacement shakes will support you on low-calorie days and keep your exercises on 'usual' days to make sure you get the foremost out of your exercise.

It is necessary to plan your calories well when pursuing this diet—on the times of fasting and non-fasting. It's suggested you usually think about: attempt to obtain a minimum of 50% of your daily calories from healthy fats like avocados, organic grass-fed milk, pastured egg yolks, copra oil, and raw nuts like macadamia, pecans, and pine nuts.

Protein: there'll be many protein—40 to 80 grams each day to stay healthy. Attempt to confirm you get your meat from organically grown, grass-fed, or pastured animals.

Fresh, organic vegetables—you should eat as many of them a day as you wish.

Pros: it is a good way to reduce. It also encourages a way healthier lifestyle as you would like to urge the foremost out of your limits on calories.

Cons: Not bingeing on 'natural' days could also be difficult. Plan ahead to assist you are doing this—setting up a food plan will assist you to continue with it.

You don't want to travel over the highest and totally undo all the great work you've done on your fasting days once you mention your non-fasting days on this plan. Once you set yourself a particular calorie limit for all days and stick with it, you'll be more successful in achieving your goals.

Food For Thought

This is sometimes mentioned because the 5:2 Fast, where regular food is consumed five days of the week, and two calories reduced fasting days.

Best for: those that need some versatility in their days of fasting. You'll easily choose your own two days every week, so you'll suit it with anything that grows up.

How it works: women can eat up to 2,000 calories per day for five days every week. On the two days of fasting, women can eat 500, but supported your BMI and level of activity; you'll get a more specific recommendation from a health care provider.

Here are some recommendations on what quite foods to eat this diet:

- Carbohydrates aren't suitable for days of fasting. They go to use most of the calories.
- Healthy calories are nuts, beans, salads, and little portions of protein.
- Used fruits, spices, and aromas to make things more exciting to eat.
- Even soups are an honest filler.
- Most people that tried the 5:2 diet found it better to skip breakfast and eat afterwards in the times of fasting. Although twiddling with eating periods is advisable to ascertain what suits you best. You'll even go from three to 2 meals.
- The best food in this diet is fresh, raw ingredients. Choose those for the tastiest food in the season.

- In case of a snack strike, have something handy at once: if you enjoy sweet things, then no-sugar jelly is ideal for fewer than ten calories.

- Drink plenty—fill up your stomach with water, tea, and occasional (remember to count the calories in milk).

- Here are some useful tips for fruit trading to assist you along the way too:

- Swap bananas in yoghurt for fresh or frozen berries for fewer than a sugar rebound.

- Replace omelette quiches or flans—all the taste, no high-calorie pastry.

- For low-fat ricotta, feta, or low-fat cheese, substitute high-fat hard cheeses.

- Replace an African-American cappuccino.

- Trade frozen dessert for home-made lollies (cordials and berries made up of low-sugar).

- Switch cauliflower rice—spray a neighbourhood of uncooked cauliflower and microwave with a lower-calorie replacement for 1-2 minutes.

- Change tagliatelle in thin ribbons with a potato peeler for 1 minute, simmer or steam, and eat together with your usual spaghetti sauce.

Pros: It can quickly change your routine, because you'll pick the two days of fasting consistent with your weekly schedule—eating the opposite days as was common, and company, socializing, and dealing out won't get in the way.

Cons: Not overeating on the 5 'natural' days is often difficult. You are going to take to make sure you do not spend calories on nutriment fixing food that will not leave you feeling full.

This is another diet that basically causes you to believe what you eat and confirm you do not lose calories. The body will enter 'repair mode' on the times of fasting, and any weakened cells inside the body are going to be restored. This intermittent pace will assist you to reap in an incredibly manageable way all the health benefits of intermittent fasting.

Spontaneous Meal Skipping

Often referred to as mini fasting, this is often a way more relaxed attitude towards fasting. It's all about understanding exactly when you're tired and when you are not, skipping meals. The strategy isn't designed or set in stone, so you'll adapt it around any schedules.

Best for: Extremely busy and stressful lifestyle people that want to fast but can't find how to blend in.

How It Works: As long as you're bound to eat well, intermittent fasting is often done by skipping meals when you're tired, not starving, or in a position to possess a rest.

The health benefits you'll get from testing this out are as follows:

- It will minimize inflammation; reduce oxidative stress and damage to the tissue.
- It will improve glucose production.
- It will boost physiological performance and body composition, including major weight decreases in obese individuals.
- LDL and overall cholesterol levels are going to be high.
- Preventing or reverse type 2 diabetes, and slowing its progression can help.
- Improving immune function and moving stem cells from inactive to self-renewal.
- It will enhance the work of the pancreas.
- It will increase levels of insulin and leptin and responsiveness to insulin/leptin.
- A lowered vital sign is going to be observed.
- Some of the cardiovascular benefits of workout are going to be replicated.
- It can help protect against disorder.
- Hazardous visceral fat levels are going to be modulated.
- It will improve the energy efficiency of mitochondrial.
- The normalization of ghrelin levels, referred to as the "hunger hormone," should improve.

- Sugar cravings are going to be reduced because the body adapts to burning fat rather than food.

- It will help to market the event of human somatotropin (HGH).

- It will improve brain-derived neurotrophic factor (BDNF) development, promote the discharge of the latest brain cells, and activate brain chemicals that protect against Alzheimer's and Parkinson's disease-related changes.

There are, as you'll see, a variety of health advantages that you simply can get from feeding when you're hungry instead of continuously grazing. Often, you'll want to ascertain thereto that you simply get a diet while you eat to remain healthy. Here are some great tips:

- Take a minimum of five servings of fruits and vegetables each day. Seek to incorporate more, if you'll.

- Increase the intake of sugar and saturated fat.

- Drink plenty of water; the recommended amount is six to eight glasses.

- Plan a minimum of two fish portions hebdomadally.

- Increase the consumption of water. Not quite 6g each day should be consumed. you'll be surprised by what proportion there's already

- Use starchy foods because of the foundation for your meals. These are working for the day as your fire.

Pros: With this diet, there's no strain. It all depends on what you think that you'll do best. The good thing about this diet is that in the least stages, you will get won't to just what you would like and wish. It can only be an honest thing to understand your body better.

Cons: it's going to take longer to ascertain results, and therefore the relaxed attitude can make it harder to stay thereto, but if you're committed enough, you'll make a true difference.

Many people find this much harder to stay too; others are suffering. Making it work for you is the most vital thing. However, if you eat healthier, this is often much simpler because food isn't full of any of the right nutrients and makes us bloated. Consuming that results in a collapse that causes us to eat more!

Natural Nightly Fasting

There is another easy fasting method, which is ideal for beginners. It's about eating at night—when we're asleep – and in the evenings. This is often a really natural method that will blend into almost any lifestyle.

Best for: Beginners—this may be a natural thanks to getting curious about fasting. Most diets recommend avoiding food in the dark; it's just a more formal thanks to doing this.

How It Works: By avoiding eating in the evenings, this is often how to fast. The sole thing you actually got to do is confirm there is a 10-

12-hour window in which you are not eating anything, including the periods you're sleeping.

The great thing about this diet is that you simply are going to be ready to maintain your exercise regime. If this is often the case, here is a few guidance on what quite a diet you'll consume while exercising:

- Low fat
- Rich in carbs and protein
- Low fibre
- Contains beverages
- Composed of common products that you simply handle well

Pros: This is often easy to show into a successful lifestyle change, which will yield results. You'll find the results much easier to take care of because it's not a strict diet.

Cons: Seeing these results can take a long, but at the end of the day, it'll be worthwhile. You'll also get to take care of what you're doing throughout the day. The more you feed, the better it'll be to stay up with this.

This diet plan comes with all the perks of intermittent fasting, without disrupting your life an excessive amount of. You'll still consume three meals each day, with the standard amount of calories you'd eat per day, nothing in the dark . it is a good way to make a go easy.

Carb Backloading

This is an intermittent fast style that helps you work out. This needs intermittent fasting and, therefore, the correct diet to make sure you retain building muscle. This is often perfect to create a healthy and lean body because it's better to enhance metabolism while retaining the muscle.

Best for: those that want to quickly build muscle. This diet reveals that fasting isn't just a matter of weight loss.

How it works: You fast for 8 hours each day, using the remaining 16 to eat. You eat all of your proteins and fats in the morning in this process, leaving most of the sugars and calories for the night after you've figured out.

Pros: This diet is ideal for bodybuilders and people who wish to do tons of labour because the fast doesn't hinder your routine and allows you to keep building your muscle efficiently.

Cons: This program takes tons of thought as you are going to possess to figure it around your exercise regime. With the right plan in situ, though, you'll see results quickly.

How does one Decide?

Determining the simplest intermittent fasting for you is essentially hooked into your eating, sleeping patterns, and job requirements. For instance, if you're employed all night, you cannot move fast in the dark because you'll be hungry; therefore, it's advisable to incorporate your fasting window into your sleeping hours. You would like to settle on an idea that works best for you. Aren't getting over-ambitious or overestimate yourself and choose a 24-hour fast on a primary day.

It will be torturous, as you would possibly find yourself eating. This may bring a sense of guilt, and most of the people tend to offer up at this stage. This is often undue to your failure; it's because you set unreasonable goals for yourself. What's most vital is to make measurable progress with reasonable goals.

Fluids to take While Fasting

While fasting, only certain fluids are often consumed like; water, tea, and occasional (hot or iced) and homemade broth.

Water

The advantages of water can't be overemphasized, so you want to drink water frequently throughout the day once you fast. You'll enjoy the flat, mineral, or soda water. you'll add;

- You can add lime
- You can add lemon
- You can add slices of other fruits (never eat the fruit or consume fruit juice)
- You can add vinegar (raw, unfiltered apple vinegar is better)
- You can add Himalayan salt
- You can add Chia and ground flaxseed (mix one tablespoon in a cup of water
- You can add sweetened powders or drops

Coffee

Consuming up to 6 cups of their caffeinated or decaf is allowed. Black coffee is preferable, but you're only allowed to feature one tablespoon of certain fats to every cup of coffee taken. You'll even have a change by taking unsweetened ice coffee. Brew your coffee, then refrigerate it or add ice cubes.

- You can add copra oil
- You can add medium-chain triglyceride oil (MCT oil)
- You can add butter
- You can add Ghee
- You can add heavy light whipping cream (35% fat)
- You can add half and half milk
- You can add milk
- You can add ground cinnamon, for flavour
- Try and avoid low fat or skimmed milk; milk is preferable
- You can add powdered dairy products
- You can add natural or artificial sweeteners of your choice

Herbal Tea

There's no limit on the amount of herb tea you'll consume in your fasting period. There is quite a number of herbal teas, which will help suppress your appetite and lower your blood glucose levels.

- Green tea: This is a superb suppressant
- Cinnamon Chai tea: This helps to lower the blood glucose levels, and it's also useful for suppressing cravings of sweet food.

- Peppermint tea: This acts as a superb suppressant. It helps with alleviating GI discomfort, like gas and bloating.
- Bitter melon tea: It helps to lower blood glucose levels
- Oolong tea: This also helps to scale back blood glucose levels

Black tea is preferable, but you're only allowed to feature one tablespoon of certain fats to every cup of coffee taken. You'll even have a change by taking unsweetened ice coffee. Brew your coffee, then refrigerate it or add ice cubes.

- You can add copra oil
- You can add medium-chain triglyceride oil (MCT oil)
- You can add butter
- You can add Ghee
- You can add heavy light whipping cream (35% fat)
- You can add half and half milk
- You can add milk
- You can add ground cinnamon, for flavour
- Try and avoid low fat or skimmed milk; milk is preferable
- You can add powdered dairy products
- You can add natural or artificial sweeteners of your choice

Homemade Broth

It's normal if you experience some lightheadedness in the primary few days of fasting. This is often caused by dehydration and low levels of electrolytes, and it can reduce by taking an honest homemade broth. Both vegetable and broth made with meat, fish, or bones will work. Bone broth is extremely beneficial because it contains an important ingredient called gelatin, which is extremely good for people that have arthritis or other joint problems. There's no limit on the quantity of broth you'll consume in the fasting day.

- You can mix any vegetable that goes above the bottom
- You can take leafy vegetables
- Carrots
- Onions or shallots
- Bitter melon
- Animal meat
- Animal bones
- Fish meat
- Fishbones
- Himalayan salt
- Any dried or fresh herbs and spices
- One tablespoon of ground flaxseed per cup
- Vegetable puree of any kind
- Potatoes, yam, beets or turnips
- Always avoid any store-bought broths albeit they're organic

Exercise In Intermittent Fasting

It might be challenging to travel from a sedentary lifestyle to a lively one. The key to growth is in small improvements daily. You'll start by going for walks, cycling, and swimming daily. You'll gradually move to resistance training and light-weight workouts. Don't start high-intensity workouts as you would like to offer your body the required time to adapt and recover.

It is important to notice that it's okay to coach on an empty stomach, but experts have advised that 45 minutes after you've got ended, your workout got to have a meal. Therefore, you'll fix your training in your eating window or start your training right before your eating window.

People believe that once you add exercise to your fast, it hinders your performance and encourages exhaustion. Research has shown that it's the other.

Increased Endurance

In a non-fasting exercise, the body makes use of glycogen for fuel, and this stops the oxidation of fatty acids. This reduces fat burning, and there's a limit on your endurance level since glycogen stores are limited in ratio to fat. When your body depends on carbohydrates for an exercise, you tend to hit a brick wall before your levels of glycogen are spent, and this slows down your physical activity. With a fasted exercise, there's no limit to which you'll reach. Fasted training increases the body's ability to burn fat for fuel, which ends up in a more profitable exercise.

Fat Adaptation and Preserved Glucose

Research has shown that fasted exercise forces the body to utilize intramyocellular lipids (fat stored in the muscle) for energy, and it increases the oxidative capacity of the muscle. In summary, a fasted exercise forces your body to use more fat instead of carbohydrates. This prevents a drop by blood glucose that happens in carbohydrate fueled exercise when the muscles use more glucose. Intermittent fasting helps the body to stimulate physiological adaptations in the muscle that ultimately results in improved exercise performance. In prolonged fast, the body produces more glucose in the primary hour of exercise while in a sparing exercise, the body relies on fatty acids and ketones. Insulin levels are reduced, and performance is optimized.

Inhibited Weight Gain

In fasted training, more fat is employed as energy, and this helps to guard against weight gain in a hyper-caloric state. Fasting exercise is simpler than fed training because it helps with the adaptations in muscles, which improves glucose tolerance and insulin sensitivity in a hyper-caloric fat-rich diet.

Intermittent Fasting for Women

Intermittent fasting, also considered IF, has now become a standard sort of weight loss. It's also said to extend energy levels, enhance motivation & stamina, also as improve cognitive performance. Although intermittent fasting seems to supply many promising benefits, it'd not be for everybody — particularly supported if you're male or female. And since it's now, more work is being conducted on intermittent fasting than for rats than humans. Whether or not intermittent fasting functions for you seems to be right down to human biology. Although smaller fasting periods are usually considered healthy for many people, women aren't recommended for a few longer fasting times linked with intermittent fasting. Intermittent fasting might be easily integrated into any lifestyle. Fasting is simply about to stop eating; thus, Intermittent fasting may be a practice in which fasting, also as eating times, is cycled. There are several trends, and most of them are influenced by personal decisions, and it can actually be harder for ladies with a family's demands.

How Is Weight Loss Difficult for Women?

When a wife and a husband attempt to live a healthy and safe lifestyle, they motivate and help each other by eating good and attending an area gym. Both works together also as do everything their general medicine doctor advises. In three months, the husband lost 10 lbs. Woman, 5. How different the outcomes are once they have performed the exact same routine. Woman have always thought that it had been easier for men to reduce, and science supports the view.

As per the Yale Journal of Biology & Medicine, female increases the danger of being overweight. Western women are 3.3 per cent more likely than their male counterparts to be overweight and three per cent more likely to be overweight. If you think about those numbers troubling, this becomes worse. The study also indicates that ladies are far more likely to die from weight-related illnesses than men. Health-related problems occur in women who have a lower BMI compared to men. Women are 6.6 times more susceptible to developing a weight-related illness than men. The factors for going far beyond exercise and diet problems and that specialize in hormonal & structural differences between men and ladies.

1. Hormones are a big weight-loss issue for ladies.

A lot of individuals lose muscle mass & gain weight once they age. The move isn't about the way calories are employed by the body, which can make weight reduction difficult. Females face one additional difficulty: menopause. Thanks to the reduction in estrogen, the postmenopausal woman is more likely to realize weight than men of equivalent age. Female hormones often store calories as fat, which takes up more room than lean muscles.

2. Being sentimental.

This is actually true: consistent with a study published in the American Journal of Clinical Nutrition in 2013, women appear to be far more emotional than men. Additionally, the reasoning behind the study was far more complicated than simply reaching bent a chocolate candy despite being nervous. Females tend to be at a lower metabolism than males. This suggests the body uses fewer calories (energy units) to work normal functions of the body, like breathing, thinking, also as flowing blood. The additional calories are stored as fat. Additionally, the human body structure usually exceeds that of males. In several other words, people would place pounds more muscle than fat, thereby raising the body mass index (BMI). Muscle, fortunately for men, consumes more calories than fat — even at rest. Women have a simple time, physiologically, hanging on to extra weight. Genetic makeup is yet one more metabolically factor which will make it harder for ladies to reduce. All of your mom & grandma had different setpoints that are theoretical weight restrictions the body is trying to stay in. Often this fixed point is moved on, which may work against the weight-loss attempts. Another trait you inherited is body shape. The study has also shown that ladies with those sorts of the body (like apple & pear) are at increased risk of being overweight or obese.

3. Metabolism.

Men and ladies have different metabolisms. Due to the upper lean muscle mass, males have a high resting rate. Because the muscle absorbs more calories than fat and doing little sometimes, the lads burn calories quite the ladies. Females store fat differently as if this wasn't enough, too. Fat has an annoying tendency for ladies to gravitate to the thighs, hips also as buttocks — areas where it's harder to lose.

Most women pursuing weight loss want immediate results. They like eliminating entire food classes or dramatically increasing caloric intake for a quicker weight loss. This approach results in nutritional yo-yo, since you already know, whereby transient effects are counteracted as that of the load returns — often even more so than before. Incremental lifestyle improvements all work to enhance safety and wellbeing. Whenever you think that why it's simpler for males to reduce, just remember: cafes sell an equivalent size of the portion, also because the bartender offers another one for everybody. It's up to you now to make a decision to stay at your specific control of the portion.

Fasting for Women's Health

Intermittent fasting is indeed a broad concept, which involves going without meals for a period of time. There are many several sorts of intermittent fasting, but typically the expected benefits are an equivalent throughout the board, like weight loss, increased strength, also as enhanced mental clarity. Few experts claim that fasting may cause a hormonal disturbance, which may cause changes in mood also as infertility, whereas others say that this is often perfectly healthy as long as you hear your body and roll in the hay correctly. Then? Let's know whether females can intermittent fast, if so, the way to roll in the hay healthily.

Is intermittent fasting safe for women?

Double board-certified doctor Amy Shah, M.D., who specialized in hormones, says it comes right down to the entire stress load. "Women are differently wired," she says, "they are wired in such how as stressful conditions on the body may have adverse effects on the hormonal cycles of girls ." Sometimes the word "stress" falls with a negative tone, but it's not all evil. There are a variety of health-promoting activities that place stress on your body, like exercise also because of the keto diet. Such activities cause positive, healthy changes in your body if you control your stress levels rightly. If you're over-stressed, though, the body won't be ready to deal with any extra stressors. in this situation, the implementation of fasting, which Shah describes, is "a hermetic stressor," to the mixture that triggers adverse hormonal changes, instead of the health benefits expected.

The bottom line is, every woman is special. With intermittent fasting, some women had the best, while others are more vulnerable to the strain it brings on the body. Though there's tons of evidence from females who have encountered everything from decreased cravings to good sleep to increased energy, there's still not enough conclusive evidence to draw definitive conclusions. What we already know needless to say, however, is that there are some classes of girls who really shouldn't be fasting. This includes someone who:

- Is pregnant or breastfeeding
- Is underweight
- Has a background of eating disorders
- Is under severe chronic stress
- Includes other big medical problems, like diabetes or high vital sign

How Can Intermittent Fast Affect The Hormones?

To know why some researchers are concerned about the security of women's intermittent fasting, it's also important to possess some information about your hormones also as how intermittent fasting may affect them. Women contain significant quantities of a compound referred to as kisspeptin, which is a particularly involved protein in reproduction — and sensitive to worry factors, like fasting. It triggers a hormone referred to as gonadotropin-releasing hormone, or GnRH when kisspeptin is released. Then GnRH triggers the discharge of FSH (or FSH) also as LH (or LH) from a brain region called the hypophyseal gland. In females, LH activates ovaries to get and emit estradiol, a mixture of estrogen and progesterone, which are two of the foremost important reproductive hormones. LH even indicates your ovaries for releasing an egg in your cycle's ovulation time. FSH promotes follicle development in the ovaries also as plays a big role in the production of estrogen. Few studies suggest that fasting reduces kisspeptin production, which in effect disrupts the event and release of estrogen & progesterone. This suggests, in theory, that certain women can undergo hormonal disturbances that cause issues like mood swings and delayed or missed periods. And this might contribute to infertility in extreme cases. But the difficulty is that much of the work into the negative effect of fasting on kisspeptin is performed on animals. One research that was performed on lambs revealed that short-term fast could reduce kisspeptin production, resulting in lower levels of LH in blood. Moreover, another research found that fasting throughout a woman's mid-follicular period had no impact on LH, FSH, estradiol, or progesterone levels — or the duration between the primary day of the cycle & ovulation, Some experts warn that fasting can trigger hormonal disruption in women, but further work is required to raised understand how human hormones are often influenced by fasting.

Can Fasting Affect Fertility?

Since fasting may have a detrimental effect on a woman's hormones, also there are fertility issues. Some health professionals think an adult female body might see fast as a risk of inevitable hunger. As a consequence, they believe the body prevents ovulation because there wouldn't be sufficient nutrition for a growing fetus to sustain. Though there are many other doctors who have contrary opinions, like Felice Gersh, M.D. Gersh states, "Depending on what we now understand; my hypothesis is that short fasting cycles would actually improve fertility." So, who is correct? Once more, the evidence isn't completely clear — and most work has been conducted on animal models, instead of on humans. Another study, however, focused at intermittent fasting in females with the polycystic ovarian syndrome, or PCOS — a disease with infertility as among the hallmark symptoms of that disorder. The finding suggests that intermittent fasting in women with PCOS could potentially boost fertility by increasing levels of glucose and insulin, IGF-1, and IGFBP1. Women with PCOS appear to possess an enhanced expression of IGF-1 & IGFBP1, two hormones that impact insulin production, consistent with the study. When insulin levels rise, it causes the body to supply more androgen hormones, like testosterone, which makes it harder to become pregnant. On the opposite hand, it's going to boost ovarian function when the insulin levels subside. Another research added to the present, claiming that restriction of short-term calories could potentially increase LH rates in women having PCOS while at an equivalent time reducing glucose, leptin, insulin & testosterone.

Intermittent Fasting and Your Period

There is also confusion about whether you'll fast in your period. But, as per Shah, if you're menstruating, you do not need to stop intermittent fasting. It's the week before matters. The week initiate to some time, Shah describes, once you are most susceptible to additional stress. That's because the amount of estrogen drops significantly, a move that also enhances your susceptibility to cortisol, the principal stress hormone. And since, as per Shah, females are hardwired to be more susceptible to external stressors, they might have detrimental effects on the body by introducing additional stress, like intermittent fasting. This doesn't automatically mean that if you're premenstrual, you would like to prevent intermittent fasting totally, but it's generally an honest idea to chop back, at least. When you're usually running a 16:8 fast schedule, you would possibly want to scale back your fast window to 12 hours every week. "And then cycle day 0 to day 14 is kind of your free pass to travel a touch further on the fast also as workouts," Shah says.

Intermittent Fasting In Menopause

Menopause is one among the most important hormonal changes in the lifetime of a lady, is another significant issue. As you reach your 50s, the mean age when menopause starts, estrogen & progesterone levels normally go down. You furthermore may subside insulin sensitive. Such hormonal changes will slow your metabolism and cause you to more susceptible to gaining weight. Often, they'll cause other unpleasant symptoms like mood swings, fatigue, brain fog, even psychological stress. This raises concerns about whether women undertaking peri- / postmenopausal should take up fast. But the fears regarding menopause & intermittent fasting are unwarranted as per Taz Bhatia, M.D., a board-certified physician with experience in women's health & hormone balance.

Bhatia considers intermittent fasting a superb method to assist you to undergo menopause pain, saying, "If you're handling weight gain, exhaustion, or insulin resistance in menopause, you would possibly want to undertake it out." In fact, you actually don't get to take her word for that. Research indicates that intermittent fasting can contribute to improving insulin sensitivity & fat loss. Researchers discovered in one particular animal study that intermittent fasting in overweight postmenopausal mice helped improve insulin tolerance, without even calorie restriction. Research also reveals that intermittent fasting may help protect the brain against stress, decrease depression, and cause increased self-esteem & achievement feelings.

Why Is Intermittent Fasting Different For Women?

Intermittent fasting means to modify in a specified schedule between the time of fasting (or avoiding both foods also as caloric drinks), and eating as was common. Surely, people, this suggests alternating days of fasting. For others, it means splitting the day into a period of fasting also as an "eating window" (e.g., feeding on noon until 6 p.m.), often referred to as time-restricted feeding. Intermittent fasting research shows promises for several positive effects, particularly when it involves diabetes prevention & improvement, obesity, heart diseases, and ageing markers. With levels of diabetes rising, research is curious about what appears to be the main influence of fasting on regulating blood glucose. Some unexpected differences have also been found, however, among intermittent fasting for men & women.

How Are Female Hormones More Affected Than Male Ones?

It would seem unfair to possess men walking around, looking fit, and ladies struggling to urge slim? Low-energy diets will make women less fertile. Becoming too slim can be a reproductive risk, and feminine physiology is exquisitely adapted to any hazards that affect fertility, and a reduced supply of food may be a major one. It makes an honest evolutionary sense because females in the mammalian universe are entirely special. Approximately all other mammals can finish a pregnancy or stop it whenever needed. In citizenry, the placenta breaches, i.e., the maternal blood vessels, also because the fetus, full control. To hoard further glucose for himself, the baby will block the action of insulin. Even the fetus can make the blood vessels dilate of the mother, changing the vital sign to possess more nutrients. Regardless of what the value to mother, the fetus is willing to exist. This mechanism, almost like the host-virus relationship by scientists, is what's considered "maternal-fetal conflict." Once a lady gets pregnant, nothing that the mother does will trigger the fetus to prevent developing. The result: Fertility could also be detrimental to both at the incorrect moment, like in a famine. That's why women's reproductive pathway is aware of multilevel metabolic energy signals.

How does the body "know"?

The hormonal balance of a female is particularly sensitive to how often, what proportion what she's eating. If there's not much to eat, then you'll reduce, and muscle is nearly the maximum amount as 25 per cent of the load loss. This is often why our approach to Soma Sciences needs adequate strength training to take care of lean muscle throughout weight loss. However, in fact, things are more complex than that. And females who aren't extremely lean may even with food shortage stop ovulating also as lose their period. For this reason, scientists have come to believe that the entire energy balance could be more critical for the hormonal cycle than that of the quantity of body fat.

Stresses & energy balance

Serious negative energy balance in females might be to stay blaming for the hormonal consequence, which occurs. So, it's not just a matter of what proportion of food you consume. A negative balance of energy in your body (taking less fuel than you actually got to cause your body to fall under energy stored; fat & muscle) may result from:

- Insufficient food
- Poor diets.
- Over-exercising.
- Over-stress.
- Illness, chronic inflammation, infection
- Too little rest & recovery

Even the intensity of trying to remain warm may utilize energy reserves. Any mixture of these stresses could also be sufficient to place you in an extreme negative energy balance, thus stop ovulation. Examples include marathon training and flu nursing;

multiple days in a row at a gym and inadequate protein & vegetables; intermittent fasting also as tension over paying the bills. Psychological stress could play an important part in destroying our hormonal balance. Our bodies can't show the difference between real danger and something fictitious created by our feelings and thoughts. The hormone cortisol hinders the hormone GnRH also as suppresses estrogen & progesterone production in the ovaries. Meanwhile, in stress, progesterone is transformed into cortisol, which means less progesterone, which results in the dominance of estrogen in the body. You'll be floating at an "obese" 30% body fat; however, if your energy balance has been negative for long enough, particularly if you're stressed, then reproduction stops. That's women's concern.

Estrogens, also as other hormones

Women appear to possess less protein, in general, than men. Women on fasts will eat much less protein. Less protein intake means taking in fewer amino acids. The activation of estrogen receptors and therefore, the synthesize insulin-like protein (IGF-1) in the liver involve amino acids. IGF-1 causes thickening of uterine wall lining also as reproductive cycle progression. Thus, low protein diets will reduce fertility. It's worth noting that estrogen is not just for a copy . Everywhere our bodies, we've estrogen receptors, even in our brains, GI tract, also as bones. Change the estrogen equilibrium, and you adjust the metabolism all over: memory, moods, digestion, healing, protein synthesis, bone formation, etc. Estrogen functions in a few ways whenever it involves appetite & energy state. First, estrogens change the peptides in the brainstem, which signal that you simply feel complete (cholecystokinin) or starving (ghrelin). Estrogens also stimulate neurons in the hypothalamus, which halt the event of appetite-regulating peptides. Do anything that triggers your estrogen to fall, and under normal conditions, you'll notice yourself feeling much hungry also as consuming tons quite you'd. Estrogens are important regulators of metabolic processes. This is often because, over time, the estrogenic metabolite ratios (estriol, estradiol, & estrone) change. Estradiol is basically the most factor, before menopause. It decreases after menopause, while estrone remains about an equivalent. It remains unclear the precise functions of these estrogens. A couple of hypothesizing that a fall in estradiol can cause fat storage increases. Since fat is getting used to making estradiol, this will actually clarify why it's harder for a few women to reduce after menopause. And it's going to function a justification for taking care of your reproductive health, albeit you are not focused on having babies.

Pregnant ladies have a clear need for extra energy. So, if you begin a family or are pregnant, it isn't an excellent idea to fast. Similarly, if you're under chronic stress, or you are not sleeping rightly, a quick will only bring more stress. Your body requires nutrients, not extra stress. If you're suffering or handling disordered eating, you'll likely know that a PEPSM procedure could take you down the trail which may cause additional issues. If you fit into any of those types, don't risk your wellbeing. Similar benefits are often experienced in some ways. If you're new exercise and diet, PEPSM may sound sort of a great weight loss strategy. Resolve your nutritional deficiencies before beginning PEPSM experiments. Confirm that first, you begin from a robust nutritional base.

Pregnancy and Intermittent Fasting

Is it OK for you to do intermittent fasting while pregnant? As was said earlier, first address your medical care physician before rolling out any delicate improvements to your eating routine and exercise caution.

There is not an outsized amount of research to offer educated suggestions on whether there are sure or negative impacts on the pregnancy. There are not many studies that checked out intermittent fasting over the whole length of pregnancy.

A large number of studies that check out pregnant women and fasting specialize in the Islamic custom of Ramadan, which lasts around 30 days. In that period, individuals fast from sunup to sundown. While pregnant and breastfeeding moms are actually free of fasting, some still keep it up with fasting.

There is a study conducted on a gaggle of girls which suggests that those that fasted in Ramadan experienced large changes in their glucose, insulin, and triglyceride levels, a bit like the opposite studies have found. A load of their children in labour was almost like the infants of girls who had not fasted.

A later study suggests these results and says that fasting for Ramadan doesn't affect childbirth. Apart from that, there was no relationship between fasting and birth. A bit like what our forefathers believed in the past; however, experts presume that more studies are required on fasting and its potential risk and impact on health.

One thing we all know is that pregnancy is the point at which you've got to focus on:

- Helping your child placed on weight
- Providing sustenance to assist with mind and body improvement
- Developing maternal fat stores if you would like to breastfeed

Significantly changing dietary patterns may inflict a scarcity of nutrients and other medical problems for both you and your child. Fasting may additionally change hormone levels.

Also, know that intermittent fasting and pregnancy manage birth weight. There's such an outsized number of other potential effects that haven't been examined - as an example, the risks, later on, affecting kids whose moms did intermittent fasting while pregnant, as an example.

Most importantly, the way fasting affects your body and pregnancy is variable and inconsistent in reference to how it's going to affect another person. Experts suggest that you simply work together with your doctor to create up some preparation for the load increase, which will happen, and every one preparation should be supported your weight (BMI) and overall wellness.

For women with BMIs in the 18.5 to 24.9 range, this usually includes being up somewhere in the measure of 25 and 35 pounds eating a good eating regimen of wholefoods and drinking tons of water. Those with more weight may have to regulate increase under the direction of an expert with cautious surveillance of their child's development.

Imagine a scenario if a lady practised intermittent fasting before pregnancy. This might seem over-exaggerated, but it's not. Ask your doctor if you're, as of now, getting too fast to ascertain what is going to work for you. It's going to be alright for you to stay fasting, just not precisely as you would possibly have thus far. Confirm to inform your medical care physician your whole history with intermittent fasting, also as your goals in continuing with it in pregnancy.

While the long-term implications aren't absolutely clear, scientists examined women fasting for Ramadan and the way it influenced things like fetal development. At the purpose when ladies had low glucose levels from fasting, it took them a usually longer amount of your time to differentiate fetal developments.

The low reappearance of fetal developments is typically determined as a notice sign you want to concentrate to, specifically, as you draw nearer to your maturity. Your infant should make around ten developments inside an hour to two, and you'll already feel improvements inside half an hour.

With confining eating to specific windows or days, it's going to be hard to urge the perfect measure of food once you are eating. This could be problematic if your child is pulling from your food storage too.

Issues like low iron are quite common for pregnant women. What's more, when a toddler doesn't get enough iron, especially in the trimester - they'll be at increased risk of getting ill before their first birthday. This is often alarming but fortunately getting good foods causes these risks to decrease.

To prevent weight, increase consistently in a healthy way, most girls should target to consume 300 extra kcals a day. That's a touch extra - sort of a glass of skimmed milk and an enormous piece of a sandwich - yet absolutely not the "eating for two" you'll have heard before you bought pregnantly.

Exercise is another piece of the circumstance. You'll feel cruddy - particularly in the trimester - however, moving your body may lower your hazard of gestational diabetes, help to extend your physical performance, and lessen your chances of needing a cesarean.

If you've exercised before pregnancy, it'll be truly amazing! Ask whether you've got to manage your daily schedule and continue onward. Just in case you're new workouts, specialize in getting around half-hour a day of sunshine exercises, like strolling, swimming, or cycling.

Shouldn't something be said about intermittent fasting and attempting to urge pregnant? At the instant, for a few entirely cool news, studies show there is a "commonly useful" tie between the way of eating and fertility. Intermittent fasting may have some influence on fertility in women with polycystic ovary disorder (PCOS). In one ongoing study, women with weight and PCOS who skipped meals usually saw an expansion in their hormonal levels, which is crucial for aiding in ovulation.

Other data suggest that weight reduction of 5 to 10 per cent may help with reproduction. Since intermittent fasting may help here, even as with insulin opposition and other medical problems, it's plausible that fasting may "progress" the richness and soundness of the physical body.

It's not a sensible idea to dive into fasting in pregnancy - particularly if you haven't tried it before. Luckily pregnancy doesn't keep going forever, and you'll attempt this system for eating to urge fitter after you give birth. (If you are doing plan to try it, ask your medical care physician first - who could possibly be your BFF at now, especially if you're breastfeeding.)

What's more, if you're feeling overpowered, always seek help. Your doctor will follow your weight at all of your pre-birth arrangements. Discuss your interest in your goals to see whether or not they have proposals to help you with downsizing - if necessary - in a way that keeps both you and child safe and healthy.

Making Intermittent Fasting Effective for ladies

Suppose you've got to undertake intermittent fasting, attempt to make sure that you catch on smartly & safely. Below are some techniques to urge you started: start with a shorter fasting window, and gradually build up.

The crux of the matter is that each woman is exclusive . Some females are more susceptible to possible negative hormonal changes in fasting, particularly those under severe stress. As compared, some women succeed with intermittent fasting.

Among the foremost powerful ways of deciding which group you belong to is to travel on your own intermittent fasting to ascertain how you are feeling. Once you notice something is wrong, it is a sure indication that your body's not responding well to the additional stress. You'll continue the plan if you are feeling fine.

Sticking to an intermittent fasting plan are often difficult. The subsequent suggestions will help people stay the course and reap intermittent fasting benefits: stay hydrated.

- Drink many water & calorie-free drinks, like herbal teas, all day long.
- Avoid obsessions with food. Schedule many ways on fasting days to prevent brooding about food, like trying to catch abreast of paperwork or watching a video.
- Rest and relax. Avoid strenuous tasks on days of fasting, while light exercise like yoga is often beneficial.
- Having a record of each calorie. If the program chosen requires any calories in times of fasting, choose nutrient-rich foods that are high in protein, fibre & healthful fats. Beans, lentils, fish, eggs, nuts
- as well as avocado are some examples.
- Eat quite voluminous foods. Prefer to fill however low-calorie foods like popcorn, raw vegetables & high-water fruits, like grapes or melon.
- Raise your taste without all the calories. Generously season the meals with herbs, spices, garlic, or vinegar. Such foods are relatively low in calories and filled with flavours, which will help to attenuate hunger feelings.

- After the fasting time, select the nutrient-dense foods. Eating high-fibre foods, high in vitamins, minerals also as other nutrients helps balance blood glucose levels and avoid nutritional deficiencies. A healthy diet also can improve weight loss for better health.

There are some important considerations to recollect before you begin the Intermittent Fasting Tour.

Caloric Consumption

With fewer hours to eat food, you're likely to consume fewer calories and, as discovered earlier, women's bodies are more susceptible to calorie restriction. Therefore, taking a more casual approach to IF, starting slow also as taking note of your body is vital. Take an interruption and consult your doctor if you notice any of the intense side effects, including a missed period or excessive fatigue. A doctor may advise on the simplest solution to your particular situation or suggest alternate means of achieving your losing weight or dietary goals.

Diet Quality

Intermittent fasting would by no means be such how out of a poor diet. Nutrient deficiencies when not having sufficient macronutrients (carbohydrates, fat, and protein) or micronutrients (minerals and vitamins) are far more common in women and particularly young women in childbearing age, and thus are related to poor dietary choices. Getting a nutritious, healthy diet is the secret to avoiding certain adverse effects of fasting while doing intermittent fasting. Once you are uncertain what to eat to satisfy your weight, loss goals with a healthy diet, yet still, try our 21-Day IF hotel plan . Prepared for your particular age, physical activity level & body target in conjunction with Registered Dietitians, it guarantees you fulfil your macro & calorie needs every day.

Index Weight & Body Mass (BMI)

Research shows that when watching adverse effects & advantages of Intermittent Fasting, it is necessary to differentiate between different body weights. Obese and overweight patients with Intermittent Fasting are making major changes. Conversely, women with average weight didn't receive equivalent metabolic benefits across the board. Underweight females should be especially careful to do intermittent fasting. And if you do not get to lose some weight, you'll also reap other Fasting advantages like cell regeneration, higher energy levels, and lower blood glucose levels. But, ensuring you've got a healthy diet and adequate caloric intake is vital to stop the side effects of intermittent fasting.

However, you want to definitely consult your doctor if you:

Are underweight or trying with weight gain. Your feeding window is going to be much shorter, meaning consuming the exact same amount or maybe more calories would be harder than usual.

Are pregnant or nursing. In this point, you'll be more careful about your lifestyle and diet.

Are under age 18 years. The results of intermittent fasting in times of rapid climb, as an example, for youngsters and adolescents, aren't alright studied, so you ought to take care of it.

Have endured from disordered eating. Restricting eating periods may raise the likelihood of getting back to old habits in disorder.

Have type 1 diabetes. IF increases insulin sensitivity, and it can influence how often insulin medication you need.

And this is often important, as a lady, to gradually ease in Intermittent Fasting.

Sudden changes in diet & lifestyle may result in many side effects like energy loss, headache, sleeping problems, rapid mood swings, and lots of others.

Mistakes Women Do In Intermittent Fasting

Intermittent fasting isn't a diet but a selected eating pattern. In recent years, this type of eating program has gained tremendous popularity, particularly for ladies above 50. you'll be fasting for 16 hours then eating over an 8hour period. It's the plan 16-8, which is additionally considered the norm. Many of us are following an every-other-day schedule at some point with extremely low caloric consumption and a traditional amount subsequent day. The way you engage in intermittent weight-loss fasting is legendary for a purpose — it functions when it's correctly performed. The utilization of intermittent fasting has many possible health benefits. A couple of advantages may include decreased cancer risk, diabetes risk, and a heart condition. It also can cause autophagy that's known to help in dementia. Whether you're using one among those approaches or another sort of intermittent fasting, avoiding the pitfalls which will hinder your efforts is vital. The subsequent are many intermittent fasting mistakes that are often made by many beginners.

Have numerous Changes Too Rapidly.

You're preparing to start out anything new, so you're excited about reaping all the benefits as soon as possible. It's normal that you simply want to immerse yourself right in. But making too many adjustments too fast could ruin your efforts. The key is to start gradually by inserting a couple of modifications at a time. As an example, if you've got planned to do two 500 calorie days per week while the opposite five eating a traditional number of calories, consider beginning with just one 500 calorie day. You ought to add the second day to your schedule after only a couple of weeks.

Not Watch the intake of liquid.

Staying in a state of fasting might be hindered even once you aren't eating. Most liquids breakfast and minimize any advantages considerably. And if they're fat also as calorie-free, drinking diet soft drinks isn't a sensible idea. Also, sweeteners with zero calories may have harmful effects on your levels of insulin. Water is that the primary liquid that you simply should be consuming in your fast. A small quantity of coffee isn't getting to kill your fast, as per Healthline. However, you are going to be taking your coffee black. The only small amount of sugar in the coffee or lime in the water will affect the time of fasting.

Not Drinking Enough Water.

While it's essential to not have the incorrect beverages while fasting, ensuring you drink tons of water is simply as important. Not having enough water will cause you to starve, and sometimes it is easy to confuse hunger for your thirst. People seem to be getting much water from the spread of the food they eat. International Food Information claims 20% of the water that our bodies are using comes from food. Meaning you'd got to intake about 20% more water than normal if you're not consuming for several hours to hide the difference.

Eating Unhealthy Foods.

Because intermittent fasting isn't a diet program, there are not any off-limits foods. This will cause many of us to fall under Hell of filling abreast of unhealthy food or getting to the fast-food drive-thru the instant the fast is up. Aren't getting willing to eat bad, if you think the fasting compensates for it. Draw up an inventory of all the nutritious foods you're keen on. Do daily grocery shopping, and remain informed while choosing food. Although fulfilling a craving with many less-than-healthy snacks is okay occasionally, eating as healthy as possible is required for optimal health & weight loss progress. The Mayo Clinic finds out that consuming healthy stuff is vital so as to make the foremost of each weight loss program. Foods that are rich in calcium, protein, and B-12 must be high on the priority list, particularly for ladies over 50 years.

Over-eating after every fast.

It is probably the best shortcoming for both beginners and people who are intermittent fasting for a few time. Using intermittent weight-loss fasting may backfire if your numerous intake calories in the eating period. A method to stop overeating is to eat greater amounts of healthier foods in eating time. This may include many fresh vegetables also as healthy salads. Being prepared by preparing menus and getting ingredients available before the fast ends is additionally a sensible idea. You are not inclined to grab something just this manner. It's important to understand that it'll take up about fortnight before you've got adapted to the extent that after whenever of fasting, you are doing not feel as hungry.

Attempt to stay to the wrong Plan.

There are several alternative ways to integrate intermittent fasting into your routine. As an example, if your fasting schedule doesn't involve eating a day from 8 pm until noon, and you've got a busy job that begins early morning, that's obviously not the right strategy for you. What fits one person won't work for anyone else as effectively. You would like to experiment a touch with various sorts of plans to realize the foremost advantages of intermittent fasting. It's fine if choosing the right strategy that works for you takes multiple weeks or more.

Exercising Too Much or Too Little.

Staying physically active is vital. You do not want to overdo it, though, particularly when you're fasting. Many newcomers may feel stressed at the start of a replacement eating plan and should miss the workout. Others could be so happy they'll overdo it. Choosing a moderate exercise routine may be a good option, particularly when starting out. You'll quickly add mild exercise to your daily routine by going for a walk with a dog for 20 minutes or ride your bike to do work.

Top Intermittent Fasting Tricks

Here are some tips and tricks for ensuring that you simply have a successful fast:

- Drink much water– as a lady; you ought to drink 1.5-2 litres per day. Confirm you drink water very first thing in the morning.
- To keep your hunger cornered, drink coffee and tea as caffeine may be a normal suppressant.
- Stay busy and do meaningful work. The busier you're, the lesser time you'll believe food. Get out of your house wherever you can!
- Get your best work finished in the morning because you are going to be the foremost inspired and have tons of energy.
- Keep it adjustable for you–the best thanks to doing that is to fast at your own speed, because the fast suits together with your lifestyle, you're more likely to stay thereto. Switch the diets around until you discover the right one.
- For a minimum of 3 weeks, provides it with an honest try- don't hand over too quickly. This makes your body to adapt that quantity of your time.
- Use vitamins for your benefit.

- Try to delay the breakfast to ascertain how long it can last. It can provide you with a transparent example for the simplest times to fast and eat.

- Don't mention you're fasting to strangers–the fewer people you meet, the less' helpful thoughts' you're forced to listen to. With you, you're doing this. Don't believe that.

- Don't forget to take advantage of coaching. Weight training to assist build up your body, which successively increases your metabolism.

- Protein can be a friend of yours. When necessary, include it in each meal and also use vitamins to assist you out.

- Eat well. Don't eat garbage on your non-fasting days. At the end of the day, this may discourage you. It's important to recollect that for the rest of the day, the primary meal of the day will set the tone. Make it an honest one!

Insider Tips For Breaking a quick

It's important to understand when to prevent fasting because it is the key to safety. If you are feeling 'real hunger', this suggests you would like to concentrate on the body and reading the signals when you're done.

The dictionary describes hunger as "the unpleasant feeling of exhaustion induced by the necessity for food." If they're not eaten at their normal mealtime, certain people are irritable, nervous, or disoriented. Others have the sensation of hunger as lightheaded, flat, weak, headachy, or hollow. Sometimes a feeding episode is caused by a growling stomach. Many of us eat once they become sad. Some, when tired, lose their appetite. External stimuli, also as emotional and physical stimuli, are plentiful, but few of them are hungry, just another burden on your system.

Other signs it's time to finish the fast include:

- Sudden sickness or nausea
- Diarrhoea
- Rapid increase or decrease in your pulse
- Excessive dehydration
- Sudden excessive weakness
- Normally, your experience may be a great indicator, often when the time is up, you'll know.

The recovery time for breaking a quick is estimated to be around four days. In this point, easy-to-digest food consumption is vital to your whole system so as to urge the new routine.

Include suggestions for stuff you ought to consume (start adding new items from the highest of the list):

- Fruit and vegetable juices
- Raw fruits
- Vegetable or bone broths

- Yoghurt (or other living, cultured milk products), unsweetened
- Lettuces and spinach (can use plain yoghurt as a dressing and top with fresh fruit)
- Cooked vegetables and vegetable soups
- Raw vegetables
- Well-cooked grains and beans
- Nuts and eggs
- Milk products (non-cultured)
- Meats and anything

More tips for breaking a quick successfully:

- Pay attention to the way that your body reacts to those new foods (above). Any adverse reactions are there for a reason.
- Look out for feeling full. Once you reach this, stop eating.
- Start with small, frequent meals. Eat every 2 hours approximately, while slowly progressing towards larger, more normal-sized meals.
- Always chew your food well as this aids digestion.
- Eat carefully to feature live enzymes and good bacteria into your body. Fresh, raw foods are an excellent thanks to achieving this.

Proven Tips For Managing Your Fast

Each segment will cover the sensible tips that are needed to manage your days of fasting. If you continue together with your own intermittent fasting regime, these will benefit you.

- Once you get hungry: there are hunger suppressants to assist you in getting through the fasting window

- When you get thirsty, these include coffee, sugar, green tea, cinnamon and chia seeds. Use these so as to assist you in getting through!

- The mixture of diet and exercise: this is often possible; several tests have shown that it's fine! You are going to figure out what time of day is best for your exercise after a short time.

- Getting tired or dizzy: this is often usually thanks to dehydration, so confirm you're drinking plenty. Increasing your salt intake is additionally advisable–particularly if headaches become a priority.

- I'm struggling here: the simplest thanks to avoiding abandoning is to remain busy. By getting out and doing something constructive, take your mind off food.

- I'm too busy: this will be for your benefit because your focus isn't always getting to get on food. Prepare a fast that matches the present hours of labour/commitments before this becomes troublesome. There is no reason for not doing that–particularly not that.

- I'm getting to gorge: once you've accomplished your fast, assume that it never happened and continue as normal. When time goes by, this may make it easier, and therefore, the body is going to be adapted.

- Things still crop up: that's why it is vital to organize. Clearing your calendar with important things and adapting is going to be an equivalent as how effective you're.

- Meeting with the negativity: not everyone knows the consequences of fasting, so it is best to only educate those that got to hear about it–relatives, close friends, etc. Others are getting to attempt to put you off or freak you out, stopping you from setting off.

- Maintaining the loss of weight: the fast isn't a fast fix. It is a long-term change in lifestyle which will assist you to keep the slimmer/healthier image you're keen on. It is also best to eat far better and keep this up– all the way.

- The way to keep going: you would like to relax if you are feeling tired. There's something the body is trying to inform you, and you would like to concentrate. That's why it's recommended that you simply clear your schedule at the outset.

Tips For Motivation And Success

"Ability is what you're capable of doing. Motivation determines what you are doing. Attitude determines how well you are doing it". Lou Holtz

Try to avoid the temptation to sabotage: one among the items which will make your efforts at intermittent fasting to be futile is that if you concede to the temptation of foods in your fridge or pantry. If you easily succumb to food on first sight, then it's advisable to buy every few days for groceries instead of stocking up weekly or bi-weekly. If you happen to remain together with your family, you'll ask them to cover any tempting foods far away from you.

- **Organize your fridge to make your fasting days easier:** Arrange your fasting day foods to at least one section of the fridge as this helps you to coach your eyes and mind to look for less than foods that you simply want to eat your fasting days. With time your eyes and mind won't wander everywhere, the fridge watching foods you are not allowed to eat.

- **Socializing doesn't need to involve food**: Food is one among the items that unite family and friends, and it's embedded in our culture. No matter this, there are other fun things that you simply can do on your fasting days that does not involve food once you are out there socializing. By concentrating on those activities, you'll take your mind off food but take care in order that you do not become a hermit while fasting.

- **If you're a trigger eater, attempt to overcome such triggers**: Everyone has something that triggers us to eat. For examples; in break time at work, you'll be triggered to travel to the slot machine while watching TV you'll want to possess a drink or some snack, or even you choose leftovers while clearing the dishes; no matter what the trigger is you've got to seek out how to beat such triggers. Before you start together with your intermittent fasting, confirm to notice all the days you snack and find how to affect those triggers. In your break time at work, you'll plan to choose a ten-minute walk, have another person clear the dining table, do some needlework, cut coupons, do some stretching or chew a bit of gum while watching TV.

- **Found out a gift system**: the simplest thanks to complete a serious goal is to line smaller goals and celebrate them once you have achieved it. Once you complete a group of fasting days, otherwise you lose a pound, you'll give yourself a touching treat. You'll buy yourself a replacement book, get a manicure, watch a movie with a beloved at the cinema or hang around by yourself at the park.

- **Get your family and friends to hitch you on your intermittent fasting plan**: Let your family and friends realize the intermittent fasting plan you would like to start and provides them with the rules. Albeit they do not partake in the program, they will offer you words of encouragement and motivation by telling you ways great you look or not exposure at your house with foods that you simply have stopped eating.

- 6. **Find a partner**: If can find a partner to intermittent fast with you, it can function an honest source of motivation. Find a family or friend that might like to try the 5:2 fast diet in order that you'll mutually support and encourage one another.

- **Don't rush**: Learn to take it at some point at a time: Don't overthink about how you'll survive the month as this will overwhelm you. you'll attempt to consider it like this, "I do not have to stay to my diet tomorrow; I just need to get through today." Say this to yourself a day, and you'll get through it.

- **Understand your body**: If you tell the difference between hunger and other feelings, you'll avoid mindless eating. Most of our mindless eating happens because we are angry, bored, or tired. Attempt to study your feelings any time you are feeling like grabbing a snack. To take your mind off it, you'll either attempt to ask your friend on the phone or attend bed.

- **If you are feeling the urge to eat attempt to drink some water**: it'd be tough to inform the difference between thirst and hunger, but anytime you are feeling the urge to urge a snack, attempt to drink a glass of water. You'll be surprised that the urge to eat may disappear more often than not.

7-Day Meal Plan

You can use the subsequent hotel plan below, but confirm to align it to the type of plan you'll implement, like 16:8 or 5:2. If you're doing the 16:8 fasting plan, you'll only consume the primary half the meals because you'll get to set a window of 8 hours per day for food consumption while the remaining hours are dedicated to fasting. You'll eat the meals from breakfast up to lunch or lunch to evening or either of the two. Just confirm that it's in the eight-hour time-frame.

On the opposite hand, if you're doing a 5:2 diet, what you ought to do is to omit two days from the hotel plan (any days will do) as you would like to eat normally for five days. The meals on the remaining two days should be modified by reducing your consumption so it'll meet the five hundred to 600 calories each day. If you're not currently fasting, you'll use the hotel plan as is with none modifications.

Day 1 (1316 Calories)

Breakfast: Deviled Eggs

Cook Time: 20 minutes

Servings: 6

Ingredients:

- 8 oz. full-fat cream cheese, softened at room temperature

- 12 eggs

- 2 tablespoons everything bagel seasoning

- ½ teaspoon salt

- 1 grind black pepper

Instructions:

- Add eggs to cold water, bring back a boil and cook for 10 minutes. Drain and increase cold water, let rest for 1-2 minutes. Peel the eggs.

- Cut eggs in half lengthwise and scoop out the yolks. Add yolks to the bowl.

- Slice cheese and increase the bowl with yolks. Blend well. Add in the salt and pepper and beat well.

- Fill egg whites with the yolk mixture. Add seasoning son top. Serve.

Nutritional info (per serving): Calories 277; Total fat 22.6 g; Saturated fat 10.5 g; Protein 14.9 g; Total carbs 3.3 g; Net carbs 3.1 g; Fiber 0.2 g; Sugar 1.6 g

Lunch: Caesar Salad with Chicken

Cook Time: 15 minutes

Servings: 4

Ingredients:

- 2 chicken breasts, grilled
- 1 head Romaine lettuce, chopped
- 2 cup grape tomatoes, halved
- Parmesan cheese strips
- For the Dressing:
- 3 garlic cloves, minced
- ½ lemon, juiced
- 1½ teaspoon Dijon mustard
- ¾ cup mayonnaise
- 1½ teaspoons anchovy paste
- 1 teaspoon Worcestershire sauce
- Salt and pepper, to taste

Instructions:

- Mix all the dressing ingredients in a bowl and whisk well to mix. Cover and refrigerate the dressing.
- In a bowl mix grape tomatoes, romaine lettuce and cooked chicken. Crumble the cheese crisps into smaller pieces. Add dressing on top.
- Toss to mix and serve.

Nutritional info (per serving): Calories 400; Total fat 25 g; Saturated fat 12 g; Protein 33 g; Total carbs 9 g; Net carbs 5 g; Fiber 4 g; Sugar 4 g□

Snack: Coconut Chocolate Chip Cookies

Cook Time: 30 minutes

Servings: 6

Ingredients:

- ¾ cup coconut, shredded
- 1¼ cups almond flour
- 1 teaspoon baking powder
- ½ cup butter (softened)
- ½ cup Swerve sweetener
- ½ teaspoon vanilla extract
- 1 egg
- ½ cup chocolate chips, sugar-free
- ½ teaspoon salt

Instructions:

- Preheat the oven to 325°F and line a baking sheet with parchment paper.
- In a bowl mix coconut with almond flour, leaven, and salt.
- Mix butter with sweetener in a separate bowl. Hammer in egg and vanilla. Stir to mix. Add this mixture to the flour mixture and hammer in well. Add in the chocolate chips.
- Shape the dough into 1½-inch balls. Place on the baking sheet 2 inches apart. Press each ball to ¼-inch thick.

- Bake for quarter-hour. Remove from the oven and funky completely. Serve.

Nutritional info (per serving): Calories 268; Total fat 17.4 g; Saturated fat 10.3 g; Protein 12 g; Total carbs 13 g; Net carbs 12 g; Fiber 1 g; Sugar 10 g☐

Dinner: Balsamic Chicken with Roasted Vegetables

Cook Time: 30 minutes

Servings: 4

Ingredients:

- 10 asparaguses, ends trimmed and cut in half
- 8 boneless, skinless chicken thighs, fat trimmed
- 2 bell peppers, sliced into strips
- ½ cup carrots, sliced into half long and cut into 3-inch pieces
- 1 red onion, chopped into large chunks
- ¼ cup + 1 tablespoon balsamic vinegar
- 5 oz. mushrooms, sliced
- 2 tablespoons olive oil
- ½ tablespoon dried oregano
- 2 sage leaves, chopped
- 2 garlic cloves, smashed and chopped
- ½ teaspoon sugar
- 1½ tablespoons rosemary

- 1 teaspoon salt

Black pepper, to taste Cooking spray

Instructions:

- Preheat the oven to 425°F.
- Season chicken with salt and pepper and spray two large baking sheets with cooking spray.
- Mix all the ingredients in a bowl and blend well. Place everything on the prepared baking sheet and spread in a single layer.
- Bake for 25 minutes. Serve.

Nutritional info (per serving): Calories 450; Total fat 17 g; Saturated fat 3 g; Protein 48 g; Total carbs 15 g; Net carbs 4 g; Fiber 11 g; Sugar 2 g□

Day 2 (1358 Calories)

Breakfast: Cream Cheese Pancakes

Cook Time: 15 minutes

Servings: 2

Ingredients:

- 2 eggs
- 4 oz. cream cheese

- ½ teaspoon baking powder
- ¼ cup almond flour
- ¼ teaspoon fine salt Cooking spray

Instructions:

- Mix eggs, flour, cheese, leaven, and salt in a blender and blend until smooth.
- Heat a frypan over medium heat and grease with cooking spray. Add 3 tablespoons batter. Cook for 3 minutes. Flip and cook for two more minutes. Transfer to a plate.
- Repeat with the remaining batter. Serve.

Nutritional info (per serving): Calories 329; Total fat 30.2 g; Saturated fat 16.7 g; Protein 10.1 g; Total carbs 5.4 g; Net carbs 4.2 g; Fiber 1.3 g; Sugar 2.9 g

Lunch: Thai Beef Salad

Cook Time: 15 minutes

Servings: 4

Ingredients:

- 1½ lb. flank steak
- 1 tablespoon olive oil
- 1 teaspoon sea salt
- 1 cup cucumbers, chopped

- 1 head lettuce, chopped
- 1 cup grape tomatoes, halved
- ¼ cup basil, cut into ribbons
- ¼ cup cilantro, chopped
- ¼ cup red onion, sliced
- ¼ cup olive oil
- ¼ cup coconut amines
- 1 tablespoon fish sauce 2 tablespoon lime juice
- 1 tablespoon Thai red curry paste

Instructions:

- Mix oil, coconut amines, fish sauce, juice, and curry paste in a bowl and whisk to mix.
- Season steak with salt on all sides. Put steak slices in a single layer into a glass baking dish. Add half the marinade over the steak.
- Cover meat with wrapping and refrigerate for 8 hours. Cover the reserved dressing and refrigerate.
- Mix lettuce, cucumbers, grape tomatoes, cilantro, red onion, and basil in a bowl. Cook beef in a hot pan until brown on all sides. Let beef rest for five minutes. Slice against the grain.
- Serve salad with beef and dressing.

Nutritional info (per serving): Calories 426; Total fat 26 g; Saturated fat 14.2 g; Protein 38 g; Total carbs 8 g; Net carbs 7 g; Fiber 1 g; Sugar 2 g☐

Snack: Buffalo Chicken Sausage Balls

Cook Time: 40 minutes

Servings: 12 balls

Ingredients:

- 3 tablespoons coconut flour
- 24 oz. bulk chicken sausage
- 1 cup cheddar cheese, shredded
- 1 cup almond flour
- ½ cup Buffalo wing sauce
- ½ teaspoon cayenne
- 1teaspoon salt
- ½ teaspoon pepper
- 2 garlic cloves, minced
- 1 teaspoon dried dill
- ⅓ cup mayonnaise
- ⅓ cup almond milk, unsweetened
- ½ teaspoon dried parsley
- ¼ cup bleu cheese, crumbled
- ½ teaspoon salt

- ½ teaspoon pepper

Instructions:

- Preheat the oven to 350°F and line 2 baking sheets with parchment paper.
- Mix cheddar, sausage, almond flour, coconut flour, buffalo sauce, cayenne, salt, and pepper in a bowl and mix well until combined.
- Roll the mixture into 1-inch balls and place on the baking sheets 1 inch apart. Bake for 25 minutes.
- Mix mayo, almond milk, garlic, parsley, dill, salt, and pepper in a bowl. Mix well and add bleu cheese in. Mix well.
- Serve balls with the sauce.

Nutritional info (per serving): Calories 255; Total fat 19.3 g; Saturated fat 4.7 g; Protein 15.3 g; Total carbs 4.2 g; Net carbs 2.5 g; Fiber 1.7 g; Sugar 5 g□

Dinner: Low Carb Chili

Cook Time: 40 minutes

Servings: 6

Ingredients:

- 1 bell pepper, chopped
- 1¼ lb. ground beef
- 8 oz. tomato paste

- 1½ tomato, chopped

- 2 celery sticks, chopped

- ½ cup onion, chopped

- 1½ teaspoons cumin

- ¾ cup of water

- 1½ teaspoon chilli powder

- 1½ teaspoons salt

- ½ teaspoon pepper

Instructions:

- Cook the meat in a frypan until brown. Drain the surplus fat and season meat with salt.

- Add peppers and onions to the pan and cook for two minutes. Mix onions, cooked meat, peppers, tomatoes, water, celery, and ingredient in a pot.

- Add the spices to the pot. Bring back a boil and reduce the warmth to low-medium. Cook for two hours while stirring every half-hour. Serve.

Nutritional info (per serving): Calories 348; Total fat 28.8 g; Saturated fat 8.5 g; Protein 14.9 g; Total carbs 7.2 g; Net carbs 5.2 g; Fiber 2 g; Sugar 3.3 g□

Day 3 (1471 Calories)

Breakfast: Oat-Free Porridge

Cook Time: 5 minutes

Servings: 1

Ingredients:

- 2 tablespoons unsweetened coconut, shredded
- ½ cup of water
- 2 tablespoons hemp hearts
- 2 tablespoons almond flour
- 1 tablespoon chia seeds
- 1 tablespoon golden flaxseed meal
- ¼ teaspoon granulated stevia
- ½ teaspoon pure vanilla extract
- 1 pinch salt

Instructions:

- Add all ingredients except vanilla to a saucepan.
- Cook over low heat for five minutes, stirring constantly. Add in the vanilla. Serve.

Nutritional info (per serving): Calories 453; Total fat 36 g; Saturated fat 10 g; Protein 18 g; Total carbs 15 g; Net carbs 5 g; Fiber 10 g; Sugar 1 g

Lunch: Caprese Zucchini Noodle Pasta Salad

Cook Time: 15 minutes

Servings: 8 cups

Ingredients:

- 8 oz. mozzarella pearls
- 1 oz. basil, chopped
- 4 zucchinis, spiralized
- 4 oz. cherry tomatoes, sliced in half
- 3 tablespoon red wine vinegar
- ¼ cup extra virgin olive oil
- 1 tablespoon lemon juice
- ¼ teaspoon garlic powder
- ½ teaspoon salt
- ¼ teaspoon pepper

Instructions:

- Whisk red wine, oil, lemon juice, garlic powder, salt, and pepper in a bowl.
- Add the remaining ingredients to a bowl and add dressing on top. Toss well to combine. Serve.

Nutritional info (per serving): Calories 186; Total fat 13 g; Saturated fat 4 g; Protein 7 g; Total carbs 4 g; Net carbs 3 g; Fiber 1 g; Sugar 3 g

Snack: Bacon and Guacamole Fat Bombs

Cook Time: 45 minutes

Servings: 6

Ingredients:

- ¼ cup butter (softened)
- ½ avocado
- 2 garlic cloves, crushed
- ½ small white onion, diced
- 1 small chilli pepper, finely chopped
- 1 tablespoon lime juice
- 2 tablespoons cilantro, chopped
- 4 slices bacon
- ¼ teaspoon sea salt Black pepper

Instructions:

- Preheat the oven to 375°F and line a baking tray with baking paper. Place the bacon strips on the baking tray.
- Bake for quarter-hour. Remove the tray from the oven and let cool. Crumble the bacon.
- Cut avocado in half, remove Hell and peel it. Add butter, avocado, chilli pepper, cilantro, crushed garlic, and lime juice to a bowl. Season it with salt and pepper. Mash with a fork until combined.

- Add onion and blend. Add bacon grease from the baking tray and blend well. Cover with foil and refrigerate for a half-hour

  .

- Shape the guacamole mixture into six balls. Roll each ball into the bacon pieces and place on a tray. Serve.

Nutritional info (per serving): Calories 156; Total fat 15.2 g; Saturated fat 6.8 g; Protein 3.4 g; Total carbs 2.7 g; Net carbs 1.4 g; Fiber 1.3 g; Sugar 0.5 g□

Dinner: Cheesy Tuna Pesto Pasta

Cook Time: 25 minutes

Servings: 4

Ingredients:

- 4 cups zucchini noodles, spiralized, cooked
- 1 cup cheddar, grated
- 1 cup yellowfin tuna in olive oil
- 7 oz. basil pesto
- 1½ cup punnet cherry tomato halved

Instructions:

- Mix pesto and tuna with oil in a bowl. Mash well. Add in ⅓ of the cheese and add all the tomatoes.

- Add noodles to the bowl, toss well to coat. Transfer the mixture to a baking dish and add the remaining cheese on top.
- Broil the dish for 4 minutes. Serve.
- Nutritional info (per serving): Calories 696; Total fat 27 g; Saturated fat 11 g; Protein 40 g; Total carbs 14 g; Net carbs 10 g; Fiber 4 g; Sugar 5 g

Day 4 (1521 Calories)

Breakfast: Keto Breakfast Bowl

Cook Time: 30 minutes

Servings: 1

Ingredients:

- 1 egg
- ¼ cup cheddar cheese, shredded
- 2 cups radishes
- 3½ oz. ground sausage
- ¼ teaspoon pink Himalayan salt
- ¼ teaspoon black pepper

Instructions:

- Cook sausage in a pan over medium-high heat until done. Remove sausage the pan and put aside.

- Cut radishes into small pieces and increase the pan. Season well. Cook radishes for 12 minutes.
- Fry the egg the way you would like and put aside. Layer the radishes with sausage on a plate, top with egg and cheese. Serve.

Nutritional info (per serving): Calories 617; Total fat 49 g; Saturated fat 11.1 g; Protein 32 g; Total carbs 7 g; Net carbs 4 g; Fiber 3 g; Sugar 5 g

Lunch: Kale and Brussels Sprout Salad

Cook Time: 15 minutes

Servings: 8

Ingredients:

- ½ lb. Brussels sprouts, outer leaves and stems removed
- ½ bunch curly kale
- 6 slices cooked bacon
- ½ cup dried cranberries
- ½ cup walnuts
- 2 tablespoons lemon juice
- ⅓ cup olive oil
- ½ teaspoon garlic powder
- 1 tablespoon Dijon mustard
- ¼ teaspoon sea salt

- ¼ teaspoon black pepper

Instructions:

- Add Brussels sprouts to a blender and blend well until chopped.
- Add kale leaves thereto and pulse until shredded.
- Whisk mustard, olive oil, juice, garlic powder, salt, and pepper in a bowl until well mixed.
- Add kale and Brussels sprouts and stir to mix. Add the cooked bacon, walnuts, and cranberries in it. Toss well. Serve.

Nutritional info (per serving): Calories 192; Total fat 17 g; Saturated fat 1.6 g; Protein 6 g; Total carbs 6 g; Net carbs 4 g; Fiber 2 g; Sugar 3 g☐

Snack: Cheddar Jalapeno Meatballs

Cook Time: 45 minutes

Servings: 8

Ingredients:

- 1½ lb. ground beef
- 1 large jalapeno, sliced
- 6 oz. sharp cheddar, grated

- ½ cup pork rind crumbs 1 egg

- 1 teaspoon chilli powder

- 2 tablespoons cilantro, chopped

- 1 teaspoon garlic powder

- ½ teaspoon cumin

- 1 teaspoon salt

- ½ teaspoon pepper

Instructions:

- Preheat the oven to 375°F and line a rimmed baking sheet with parchment paper.
- Mix all ingredients in a blender. Blend on high until well combined. Roll the dough into 1½-inch balls and add to the baking sheet 1 inch apart.
- Bake for 20 minutes. Serve.

Nutritional info (per serving): Calories 368; Total fat 24 g; Saturated fat 9.7 g; Protein 33.4 g; Total carbs 1.1 g; Net carbs 0.8 g; Fiber 0.3 g; Sugar 1 g

Dinner: Keto Meatloaf

Cook Time: 1 hour

Servings: 6

Ingredients:

- 2 eggs

- 2 lbs. 85% lean grass-fed ground beef

- ¼ cup nutritional yeast

- 1 tablespoon lemon zest

- 2 tablespoons avocado oil

- ¼ cup parsley, chopped

- 4 garlic cloves

- ¼ cup oregano, chopped

- ½ tablespoon pink Himalayan salt

- 1 teaspoon black pepper

Instructions:

- Preheat the oven to 400°F. Mix beef, yeast, salt, and pepper in a bowl.

- Mix eggs, oil, garlic, and herbs in a blender and blend until everything is mixed well. Add this mixture to the beef and mix well.

- Add the meat mixture to small loaf pan. Arrange the pan on the centre rack and bake for 1 hour. Remove the pan from the oven. Let cool for 10 minutes. Serve.

Nutritional info (per serving): Calories 344; Total fat 29 g; Saturated fat 13.4 g; Protein 33 g; Total carbs 4 g; Net carbs 2 g; Fiber 2 g; Sugar 1 g□

Day 5 (1371 Calories)

Breakfast: Sausage and Peppers No Egg Breakfast Bake

Cook Time: 50 minutes

Servings: 4

Ingredients:

- 1½ teaspoon olive oil
- 1 green bell pepper, chopped
- 1 red bell pepper, chopped
- ½ cup mozzarella cheese, grated
- 10 oz. sausage
- Salt, black pepper, to taste

Instructions:

- Preheat the oven to 450°F and grease a medium-sized dish with cooking spray.
- Add peppers to the baking dish and toss with 1 teaspoon vegetable oil and add salt and black pepper on top. Bake for20 minutes.
- Heat remaining vegetable oil on a pan and add the sausages. Cook over medium-high heat for 12 minutes.

- Cut sausages into pieces. Add the sausages to the baking pan with the peppers. Bake for five more minutes.

- Remove the dish from the oven, turn the oven to broil. Add the mozzarella over the peppers and sausages. Boil for 2 minutes. Serve.

Nutritional info (per serving): Calories 246; Total fat 13 g; Saturated fat 5 g; Protein 26 g; Total carbs 5 g; Net carbs 4 g; Fiber 1 g; Sugar 2 g□

Lunch: Curried Cabbage Coconut Salad

Cook Time: 5 minutes

Servings: 4

Ingredients:

- ¼ cup of coconut oil
- ½ head white cabbage, shredded
- 1 lemon juice
- ⅓ cup dried coconut, unsweetened
- ¼ cup tamari sauce
- ½ teaspoon ginger, dried
- 3 teaspoons sesame seeds
- ½ teaspoon curry powder
- ½ teaspoon cumin

Instructions:

- Add all the ingredients to a bowl and toss well.
- Cover and refrigerate for 1 hour. Serve.

Nutritional info (per serving): Calories 309; Total fat 5 g; Saturated fat 8 g; Protein 12 g; Total carbs 12 g; Net carbs 6 g; Fiber 6 g; Sugar 3 g

Snack: Cheesy Party Crackers

Cook Time: 45 minutes

Servings: 8

Ingredients:

- ½ cup flax meal
- 1 cup almond flour
- 2 tablespoons whole psyllium husks
- 1 cup of water
- 1 cup Parmesan cheese, grated
- 1 teaspoon salt
- ¼ teaspoon black pepper

Instructions:

- Mix flax meal, almond flour, psyllium, salt, and pepper in a bowl. Add the cheese thereto and blend well. Add water and mix well. Let rest for quarter-hour.

- Preheat the oven to 320°F and divide the dough into two parts.
- Place half the dough on a parchment paper. Place another piece of parchment paper on top and roll the dough out until thin.
- Cut the dough into 16 equal pieces. Repeat the method with the remaining dough.
- Bake for 45 minutes. Serve.

Nutritional info (per serving): Calories 169; Total fat 13.4 g; Saturated fat 2.7 g; Protein 8.4 g; Total carbs 6.3 g; Net carbs 1.7 g; Fiber 4.5 g; Sugar 0.8 g□

Dinner: Crispy Salmon with Pesto Cauliflower Rice

Cook Time: 40 minutes

Servings: 3

Ingredients:

- 1 tablespoon olive oil
- 3 salmon fillets
- 1 tablespoon coconut amines
- 1 teaspoon fish sauce
- 1 tablespoon butter
- 3 garlic cloves
- 1 cup basil leaves, chopped

- ¼ cup hemp hearts
- ½ cup olive oil
- 1 lemon juice
- ½ teaspoon pink salt
- 3 cups riced cauliflower, frozen
- 1 scoop MCT powder pinch salt

Instructions:

- Add fish sauce, coconut amines, and vegetable oil to a baking dish. Pat the salmon fillets and add place into the dish, skin side down. Add a pinch of salt. Let rest for 20 minutes.
- Heat an iron skillet on medium heat.
- Peel and dice the garlic and add it to a blender. Add hemp hearts, basil, juice, olive oil, MCT powder, and salt. Pulse well to mix.
- Heat cauliflower rice in a skillet. Add pesto and pink salt. Mix well to mix. Lower the warmth and keep it warm.
- Add butter to the iron skillet placed over medium heat. Add salmon skin side down. Cook for five minutes. Flip the salmon and add the remaining marinade from the plate. Sear for two minutes.
- Remove from heat and serve on top of rice. Enjoy!

Nutritional info (per serving): Calories 647; Total fat 51 g; Saturated fat 10.8 g; Protein 33.8 g; Total carbs 8 g; Net carbs 5 g; Fiber 3 g; Sugar 3 g☐

Day 6 (1237 Calories)

Breakfast: Bacon and Egg Breakfast Muffins

Cooking time: 25 minutes

Servings: 12 Ingredients:

- 8 eggs
- 8 bacon slices
- ⅔ cup green onion, chopped
- Cooking spray

Instructions:

- Coat the muffin tin with nonstick cooking spray and preheat the oven to 350°F.
- Add bacon to an outsized pan and cook over medium heat until crisp. Transfer to a plate lined with paper towels. Let cool then chop into small pieces.
- Add eggs to a bowl and whisk well. Then add green onions and cooked bacon. Mix until everything is well combined.
- Add the mixture to the muffin tin. Bake for about 20-25 minutes, until edges are golden brown.

- Let the muffins cool and luxuriate in bacon and egg breakfast muffins.

Nutritional info (per serving): Calories 158; Total fat 13.3 g; Saturated fat 1.7 g; Protein 8 g; Total carbs 1 g; Net carbs 1 g; Fiber 0 g; Sugar 1 g□

Lunch: Grilled Chicken Salad

Cooking time: 20 minutes

Servings: 2

Ingredients:

- ½ lb. chicken thigh, grilled and sliced
- 1 teaspoon fresh thyme
- 4 cups romaine lettuce, chopped
- 2 garlic cloves, crushed
- ¼ cup cherry tomatoes, chopped
- 3 tablespoons extra virgin olive oil
- ½ cucumber, thinly sliced
- 2 tablespoons red wine vinegar
- ½ avocado, sliced
- 1 oz. olives, pitted and sliced
- 1 oz. Feta cheese, crumbled
- Salt, pepper, to taste

Instructions:

- Season chicken with a teaspoon of thyme, crushed garlic, pepper, and salt.
- Preheat oil in a pan over medium heat. Cook chicken until golden brown.
- Mix olives, sliced cucumber, chopped lettuce, sliced avocado, and ¼ cup tomatoes in a large bowl.
- Add chicken to the salad. Sprinkle with crumbled cheese.
- Drizzle with vegetable oil and vinegar. Enjoy!

Nutritional info (per serving): Calories 617; Total fat 52 g; Saturated fat 4 g; Protein 30 g; Total carbs 11 g; Net carbs 7 g; Fiber 4 g; Sugar 2.5 g☐

Snack: Keto Almond Bark

Cooking time: 15 minutes

Servings: 20

Ingredients:

- 4 oz. cocoa butter
- ½ cup Swerve sweetener
- ½ teaspoon vanilla extract
- 2 tablespoons water
- ¾ cup cocoa powder
- 1 tablespoon butter

- ½ cup powdered Swerve sweetener
- 1½ cups roasted almonds, unsalted
- 2½ oz. unsweetened chocolate, chopped
- ¼ teaspoon sea salt

Instructions:

- Add 2 tablespoons water and ½ cup Swerve sweetener to a saucepan. Bring the mixture to a light-weight boil, stirring occasionally. Cook for about 8 to 9 minutes until the mixture darkens.

- Turn the warmth off and whisk in 1 tablespoon butter. Add 1½ cups roasted almonds and toss well until coated. Then stir in 2 pinches of salt.

- Spread almonds onto a parchment-lined baking sheet. Add 4 oz. of cocoa butter and 2½ oz. of unsweetened chocolate to an outsized saucepan. Melt over medium heat and stir until smooth.

- Stir in ¾ cup chocolate and ½ cup powdered Swerve sweetener until smooth. Turn the warmth off and stir in ½teaspoon vanilla.

- Reserve 4 tablespoons of almonds and keep them aside. Add leftover almonds to the chocolate mixture and stir well.

- Spread chocolate-almond mixture out onto an equivalent baking sheet. Top with reserved ¼ cups of almonds and sprinkle with salt.

- Chill for about 3 hours then forced entry chunks. Serve right away!

Nutritional info (per serving): Calories 144; Total fat 14 g; Saturated fat 1.3 g; Protein 13 g; Total carbs 5 g; Net carbs 2 g; Fiber 3 g; Sugar 10 g □

Dinner: Chicken Parmesan

Cooking time: 19 minutes

Servings: 8

Ingredients:

- 2 lbs. boneless skinless chicken breast
- 4 oz. fresh mozzarella
- ⅓ cup sugar-free marinara
- 1 cup almond flour
- 1 cup parmesan cheese, grated
- 2 eggs
- 1 teaspoon Italian seasoning
- ½ teaspoon black pepper
- ½ teaspoon sea salt

Instructions:

- Add chicken to a bag and pound until about ½-inch thick.

- Add 1 teaspoon Italian seasoning, a cup of parmesan cheese, ½ teaspoon sea salt, a cup of almond flour, and ½teaspoon pepper. Mix well.

- Add eggs to a separate bowl and whisk well. Pat dry the chicken with paper towels.

- Dip chicken into the egg mixture then coats with almond flour mixture. Brush with oil or coat with cooking spray.

- Preheat the oven to 425°F. Place chicken on a baking sheet lined with parchment paper. Cook for about 11-12 minutes.

- Then flip the chicken, spray with cooking spray and cook for five minutes more.

- Sprinkle each bit with mozzarella and drizzle with spaghetti sauce. Transfer back to the oven and cook for a few minutes until cheese is melted.

Nutritional info (per serving): Calories 318; Total fat 17 g; Saturated fat 5 g; Protein 36 g; Total carbs 4 g; Net carbs 3 g; Fiber 1 g; Sugar 1 g☐

Day 7 (1258 Calories)

Breakfast: Chocolate Mint Avocado Smoothie

Cooking time: 5 minutes

Servings: 1

Ingredients:

- 2 scoops chocolate collagen protein
- 2 tablespoons coconut, shredded
- ½ cup of coconut milk
- 1 tablespoon cacao butter, crushed
- 1 cup of water
- 4 mint leaves
- ½ cup ice ½ a frozen avocado

Instructions:

- Add all the ingredients apart from shredded coconut and collagen protein to a blender.
- Blend on high for about 45 seconds. Then add collagen protein to a blender and blend for five seconds more.
- Top the chocolate mint avocado smoothie with coconut flakes.

Enjoy!

Nutritional info (per serving): Calories 552; Total fat 44 g; Saturated fat 25 g; Protein 26 g; Total carbs 10 g; Net carbs 1 g; Fiber 9 g; Sugar 2 g ☐

Lunch: Italian Salad

Cooking time: 15 minutes

Servings: 4

Ingredients:

- 1 cup mixed Italian olives, pitted
- 6 oz. deli ham, diced
- 6 cups Romaine lettuce, shredded
- ¼ cup pickled banana peppers, sliced
- 2 medium Roma tomatoes, diced
- ¼ red onion, sliced
- For the Vinaigrette:
- 1 tablespoon red wine vinegar
- 1 tablespoon Italian seasoning
- ½ cup olive oil
- A pinch of sea salt
- Black pepper, to taste

Instructions:

- Add all vinaigrette ingredients to a bowl and whisk well to mix.
- Arrange all the salad ingredients in a large bowl and top with the dressing. Toss well to mix. Enjoy!

Nutritional info (per serving): Calories 289; Total fat 24 g; Saturated fat 7 g; Protein 11 g; Total carbs 7 g; Net carbs 4 g; Fiber 3 g; Sugar 3 g □

Snack: Brussels Sprouts Chips

Cooking time: 15-20 minutes

Servings: 4

Ingredients:

- 1 lb. Brussels sprouts washed and dried, ends trimmed
- 1 teaspoon salt
- 2 tablespoons extra virgin olive oil
- Smoked paprika, for serving

Instructions:

- Preheat the oven to 400°F
- Peel the outer leaves of the Brussels sprouts and discard them. Add the sprouts to a bowl.
- Drizzle with oil and toss well to coat in oil. Season it with salt. Spread on a baking sheet evenly in one layer.
- Bake for about 12-15 minutes. Take them out from the oven and allow them to cool.
- Sprinkle with more salt if you would like. Serve topped with smoked paprika.
- Nutritional info (per serving): Calories 104; Total fat 7 g; Saturated fat 1.4 g; Protein 3 g; Total carbs 9 g; Net carbs 5 g; Fiber 4 g; Sugar 1 g

Dinner: Mushroom Bacon Skillet

Cooking time: 10 minutes

Servings: 1

Ingredients:

- ½ teaspoon salt
- 1 tablespoon garlic, minced
- 4 slices pastured pork bacon, cut into ½-inch pieces
- 2 sprigs thyme, leaves only
- 2 cups mushrooms, halved

Instructions:

- Preheat a skillet over medium heat. Add bacon and cook until crispy. Remove from the pan.
- Add sliced mushrooms. Sauté until softened, stirring often.
- Add garlic, thyme, and salt. Cook for five minutes more, stirring often.
- When mushrooms become golden, turn the warmth off.
- Garnish mushroom bacon with greens and enjoy!

Nutritional info (per serving): Calories 313; Total fat 8.5 g; Saturated fat 3.8 g; Protein 13.6 g; Total carbs 8.4 g; Net carbs 0.3 g; Fiber 8.1 g; Sugar 2.2 g

Intermittent Fasting Recipes

Breakfast

Zucchini Omelet

Preparation time: 4 minutes Cooking time: 3 hours and 30 minutes

Servings: 6

Ingredients:

- 1½ cups red onion, chopped
- 1 tablespoon olive oil
- 2 garlic cloves, minced
- 2 teaspoons fresh basil, chopped
- 6 eggs, whisked
- A pinch of sea salt and black pepper
- 8 cups zucchini, sliced
- 6 ounces fresh tomatoes, peeled, crushed

Directions:

In a bowl, mix all the ingredients except the oil and therefore the basil.

Grease the slow cooker with the oil, spread the omelette mix in the bowl, cover and cook on low for 3 hours and half-hour.

Divide the omelet between plates, sprinkle the basil on top and serve for breakfast.

Nutrition: calories 156, fat 7,2, fiber 4,3, carbs 16,7, protein 8,8

Chili Omelet

Preparation time: 5 minutes Cooking time: 3 hours and 30 minutes

Servings: 4

Ingredients:

- 2 garlic cloves, minced
- 1 tablespoon olive oil
- 1 red bell pepper, chopped
- 1 small yellow onion, chopped
- 1 teaspoon chilli powder
- 2 tablespoons tomato puree
- ½ teaspoon sweet paprika
- A pinch of salt and black pepper
- 1 tablespoon parsley, chopped
- 4 eggs, whisked

Directions:

In a bowl, mix all the ingredients except the oil and therefore the parsley and whisk them well.

Grease the slow cooker with the oil, add the egg mixture, cover and cook on low for 3 hours and half-hour.

Divide the omelette between plates, sprinkle the parsley on top and serve for breakfast.

Nutrition: calories 118, fat 8,2, fiber 1,3, carbs 6, protein 6,4

Basil and Cherry Tomato

Breakfast Preparation time: 4 minutes Cooking time: 4 hours Servings: 4

Ingredients:

- 1 tablespoon olive oil
- 2 yellow onions, chopped
- 2 pounds cherry tomatoes, halved
- 3 tablespoons tomato puree 2 garlic cloves, minced
- A pinch of sea salt and black pepper 1 bunch basil, chopped

Directions:

Grease the slow cooker with the oil, add all the ingredients, cover and cook on high for 4 hours. Stir the mixture, divide it into bowls and serve for breakfast.

Nutrition: calories 101, fat 4,1, fiber 4,2, carbs 15,6, protein 3

Carrot Breakfast Salad

Preparation time: 5 minutes Cooking time: 4 hours Servings: 4

Ingredients:

- 2 tablespoons olive oil
- 2 pounds baby carrots, peeled and halved
- 3 garlic cloves, minced
- 2 yellow onions, chopped
- ½ cup vegetable stock
- 1/3 cup tomatoes, crushed
- A pinch of salt and black pepper

Directions:

In your slow cooker, combine all the ingredients, cover and cook on high for 4 hours. Divide into bowls and serve for breakfast.

Nutrition: calories 169, fat 7,6, fiber 8, carbs 25,4, protein 2,3

Sweet Squash Mix

Preparation time: 5 minutes Cooking time: 7 hours Servings: 6

Ingredients:

- 6 pounds butternut squash, peeled and cut into cubes
- 1 cup apple cider
- 1 teaspoon ground cinnamon
- 1 teaspoon fresh ginger, grated
- ½ cup maple syrup
- A pinch of ground nutmeg

Directions:

In your slow cooker, mix all the ingredients, cover and cook on low for 7 hours. Divide into bowls and serve for breakfast.

Nutrition: calories 294, fat 0,6, fiber 9,4, carbs 76, protein 4,6

Balsamic Onion Jam

Preparation time: 5 minutes Cooking time: 4 hours and 15 minutes

Servings: 6

Ingredients:

- 2 tablespoons olive oil
- 4 pounds yellow onions, sliced
- ½ teaspoon baking soda
- 5 garlic cloves, minced
- ½ cup water
- ¼ cup balsamic vinegar
- 1 teaspoon dried thyme
- A pinch of salt and black pepper
- 1 teaspoon red pepper flakes
- 2 tablespoons coconut sugar

Directions:

Heat up a pan with the oil over medium heat, add the onions and bicarbonate of soda, stir, sauté for quarter-hour and transfer to a slow cooker.

Add the remainder of the ingredients, whisk, cover and cook on low for 4 hours.

Stir the jam, divide into jars and serve for breakfast or any time of day.

Nutrition: calories 176, fat 5, fiber 6,7, carbs 31,4, protein 3,6

Lunch

Turmeric Rack of Lamb

Preparation time: 15 minutes Cooking time: 16 minutes

Servings: 4

Ingredients:

- 13 oz rack of lamb
- 1 tablespoon ground turmeric
- ½ teaspoon chilli flakes
- 3 tablespoons olive oil
- 1 tablespoon balsamic vinegar
- 1 teaspoon salt

- ½ teaspoon peppercorns
- ¾ cup of water

Directions:

In the shallow bowl, misunderstanding together ground turmeric, chilli flakes, olive oil, balsamic vinegar, salt, and peppercorns. Brush the rack of lamb with the oily mixture generously.

After this, preheat grill to 380F.

Place the rack of lamb in the grill and cook it for 8 minutes from all sides.

The cooked rack of lamb should have a light-weight crunchy crust.

Nutrition: calories 252 fat 18.8, fiber 0.4, carbs 1.3, protein 18.9

Sausage Casserole

Preparation time: 10 minutes Cooking time: 35 minutes

Servings: 6

Ingredients:

- 2 jalapeno peppers, sliced
- 5 oz Cheddar cheese, shredded
- 9 oz sausages, chopped
- 1 tablespoon olive oil
- ½ cup spinach, chopped

- ½ cup heavy cream

- ½ teaspoon salt

Directions:

Brush the casserole mould with the vegetable oil from inside.

Then put the chopped sausages in the casserole mould in one layer.

Add chopped spinach and sprinkle it with salt.

After this, add sliced jalapeno.

Then make the layer of shredded cheddar.

Pour the cream over the cheese.

Preheat the oven to 355F.

Transfer the casserole in the oven and cook it for 35 minutes.

Use the kitchen torch to make the crunchy cheese crust of the casserole.

Nutrition: calories 296, fat 26, fiber 0.3, carbs 1, protein 14.5

Cajun Pork Sliders

Preparation time: 10 minutes Cooking time: 45 minutes

Servings: 4

Ingredients:

- 4 low carb bread slices

- 14 oz pork loin

- 2 tablespoons Cajun spices 1

- tablespoon olive oil

- 1/3 cup water

- 1 teaspoon tomato sauce

Directions:

Rub the cut of pork with Cajun spices and place in the skillet.

Add vegetable oil and roast it over the high heat for five minutes from all sides.

After this, transfer the meat in the saucepan, add spaghetti sauce and water.

Stir gently and shut the lid.

Simmer the meat for 35 minutes.

Slice the cooked cut of pork.

Place the pork sliders over the bread slices and transfer in the serving plates.

Nutrition: calories 382, fat 22.4, fiber 4.5, carbs 2.4, protein 38.9

Coated Cauliflower Head

Preparation time: 10 minutes

Cooking time: 40 minutes

Servings: 6

Ingredients:

- 2-pound cauliflower head
- 3 tablespoons olive oil
- 1 tablespoon butter, softened
- 1 teaspoon ground coriander
- 1 teaspoon salt
- 1 egg, whisked
- 1 teaspoon dried cilantro
- 1 teaspoon dried oregano
- 1 teaspoon tahini paste

Directions:

Trim cauliflower head if needed.

Preheat oven to 350F.

In the bowl, mix together vegetable oil, softened butter, ground coriander, salt, whisked egg, dried cilantro, dried oregano, and tahini paste.

Then brush the cauliflower head with this mixture generously and transfer in the tray.

Bake the cauliflower head for 40 minutes.

Brush it with the remaining oil mixture every 10 minutes.

Nutrition: calories 131, fat 10.3, fiber 4, carbs 8.4, protein 4.1

Artichoke Petals Bites

Preparation time: 10 minutes Cooking time: 10 minutes

Servings: 8

Ingredients:

- 8 oz artichoke petals, boiled, drained, without salt
- ½ cup almond flour
- 4 oz Parmesan, grated
- 2 tablespoons almond butter, melted

Directions:

In the bowl, mix together almond flour and grated Parmesan.

Preheat the oven to 355F.

Dip the artichoke petals in the almond butter then coat in the almond flour mixture.

Place them in the tray.

Transfer the tray in the preheated oven and cook the petals for 10 minutes. Chill the cooked petal bites little before serving.

Nutrition: calories 140, fat 6.4, fibre 7.6, carbs 14.6, protein 10

Snacks

Squash Bites

Preparation time: 10 minutes Cooking time: 40 minutes Servings: 4

Ingredients:

- 10 ounces turkey meat, cooked, sliced
- 2 pounds butternut squash, cubed
- 1 teaspoon chilli powder
- 1 teaspoon garlic powder
- 1 teaspoon sweet paprika Black pepper to taste

Directions:

In a bowl, mix butternut squash cubes with flavour, black pepper, garlic powder and paprika and toss to coat.

Wrap squash pieces in turkey slices, place all of them on a lined baking sheet, place in the oven at 350 degrees F, bake for 20 minutes, flip and bake for 20 minutes more.

Arrange squash bites on a platter and serve.

Enjoy!

Nutrition: calories 223, fat 3,8, fiber 4,5, carbs 26,5, protein 23

Zucchini Chips

Preparation time: 10 minutes Cooking time: 12 minutes Servings: 4

Ingredients:

- 1 zucchini, thinly sliced
- A pinch of sea salt
- Black pepper to taste
- 1 teaspoon thyme, dried 1 egg
- 1 teaspoon garlic powder
- 1 cup almond flour

Directions:

In a bowl, whisk the egg with a pinch of salt.

Put the flour in another bowl and blend it with thyme, black pepper, and garlic powder.

Dredge zucchini slices in the egg mix then in flour.

Arrange chips on a lined baking sheet, place in the oven at 450 degrees F and bake for six minutes on all sides,

Serve the zucchini chips as a snack.

Enjoy!

Nutrition: calories 106, fat 8,2, fiber 2,1, carbs 5,2, protein 5,1 19.

Pepperoni Bites

Preparation time: 5 minutes Cooking time: 10 minutes Servings: 24 pieces

Ingredients:

- 1/3 cup tomatoes, chopped
- ½ cup bell peppers, mixed and chopped 24 pepperoni slices
- ½ cup tomato sauce
- 4 ounces almond cheese, cubed
- 2 tablespoons basil, chopped Black pepper to taste

Directions:

Divide pepperoni slices into a muffin tray.

Divide tomato and bell pepper pieces into the pepperoni cups.

Also divide the spaghetti sauce, basil and almond cheese cubes, sprinkle black pepper at the top, place cups in the oven at 400 degrees F and bake for 10 minutes.

Arrange the pepperoni bites on a platter and serve.

Enjoy!

Nutrition: calories 59, fat 4,5, fiber 0,1, carbs 2, protein 2,5

Party Meatballs

Preparation time: 10 minutes Cooking time: 40 minutes Servings: 20

Ingredients:

- 1-pound turkey meat, ground

- 1 tablespoon coconut oil, melted

- 1 yellow onion, chopped

- 1 egg

- 1 cup coconut flour

- 1 teaspoon Italian seasoning

- A pinch of sea salt

- Black pepper to taste

- 2 tablespoons parsley, chopped

Directions:

In a bowl, mix turkey meat with half the flour, a pinch of salt, black pepper, Italian seasoning, parsley, onion, egg and sauce and stir well.

Put the remainder of the flour in another bowl.

Shape 20 turkey meatballs and dip all in flour.

Heat up a pan with the oil over medium-high heat, add meatballs, cook them for 4 minutes on all sides, transfer to paper towels to get rid of any excess grease, place all of them on a platter and serve.

Enjoy!

Nutrition: calories 71, fat 2,6, fiber 2,2, carbs 4,1, protein 7,7

Chicken Strips

Preparation time: 10 minutes Cooking time: 20 minutes Servings: 4

Ingredients:

- 1-pound chicken tenders
- 1 egg, whisked A pinch of sea salt
- 1/3 cup coconut, unsweetened and shredded
- ¼ cup coconut flour

Directions:

In a bowl, mix coconut with coconut flour and a pinch of sea salt and stir.

Put the whisked egg in another bowl.

Dip chicken pieces in egg, then in coconut mixture, arrange all of them on a lined baking sheet and bake at 350 degrees F for 25 minutes.

Serve as a snack.

Enjoy!

Nutrition: calories 330, fat 13,6, fiber 8,1, carbs 13,6, protein 36,9

Conclusion

Thanks, another time for getting this precise guide **- *Intermittent Fasting for Ladies.***

As you've seen from all the knowledge in this book, intermittent fasting will help tenfold in your life.

There are many various diets to settle on from and to suit yourself; you ought to match the fasting in with whatever time of day you're busy. And while you're doing the fast, you'll keep exercising, so there's really no reason to not provides it with a go!

There will be moments where you discover it difficult and there'll be times once you want to offer up, and this is often the safest time to hunt guidance from others who are through an equivalent thing.

To your success,

Emma Lyron